WHEN I LEARN...
SURVIVING STROKE WITH PRIDE

By

Donna Brady

*Lori,
To a wonderful friend who I enjoy spending time with! Keep up the bantering
Donna Brady*

This book is a work of non-fiction. Names and places have been changed to protect the privacy of all individuals. The events and situations are true.

© 2002 by Donna Brady. All rights reserved.

No part of this book may be reproduced, stored in a retrieval system, or transmitted by any means, electronic, mechanical, photocopying, recording, or otherwise, without written permission from the author.

ISBN: 1-4033-4280-6 (e-book)
ISBN: 1-4033-4281-4 (Paperback)

Library of Congress Control Number: 2002108004

This book is printed on acid free paper.

Printed in the United States of America
Bloomington, IN

1stBooks - rev. 06/03/03

Dedication

This book is dedicated to :
- My husband for unconditionally sticking by my side
- Christine for helping me get the simple things in life back
- My family for standing by us
- Those that cared enough to help me see it through

Contents

Dedication iii
Preface vii
Foreword ix
Chapter 1: The Stroke 1
   The first day 1
   My hospital stay: 2
   The Priest 4
   The Test 7
   The hospital therapist 10
   Two weeks later 11
   Home at last 13
Chapter 2: Therapy 15
   The first day of therapy 15
   The day my real learning began 16
   My first big assignment 19
   Lost in surgery 29
   Leaving Therapy 30
   My way to say "thank you" 35
   Testing a new life 41
   Looking at the old life 43
   The first book I read 45
   Encounter of compassion 46
Chapter 3: Emotional Rage 48
   Loss 48
   Panic 54
   Hiding 66
   Help Me 68
   Anger 77
   Depression 80
   Hope 87
Chapter 4: Relearning 90
   Work Day 1 90
   July 31, 1998 95

    Needle in a haystack..97
    Step by Step..99
Chapter 5: From My Husbands Perspective................102
Chapter 6: How kids cope...115
    How they react to the stress......................................115
    Helping or children recover.......................................117
Chapter 7: Write, Write, Write 121
    Clouds 123
    A Child's Kiss 123
    Short thoughts 124
    The Fight 129
    Reflections Feb. 20, 1998..130
    Thoughts on why...130
Chapter 8: Remembering Five Years Past...................132
    When the Spirit Found Me 133
    Instilling Change 136
Chapter 9: Kindness from the heart.............................138

Preface

Hi my name is Donna. I am a stroke survivor. I had my stroke at the age of 33 during the prime of my life. It was 6 days after the birth of my third daughter. We may never fully understand why I had a stroke or why it was to be such a big part of my life. I do know that stroke takes from you. It takes from your family and friends too but it can also give back. What I am hoping is that talking about my stroke, my recovery, and my survival will help others who are touched in someway by stroke. To help others see and feel how so many of us see and feel. My purpose is to help give a sense of hope, understanding and compassion for life and love after stroke. We all must endure pain in our lives but it is truly up to us to seek out its understanding and learn from it. Learning does not just happen you have to search for it. The harder you work, the more you understand, and the more you understand the more satisfying life after stroke can be.

Little did I know that by my thirty-fourth birthday, my life would change forever. I wrote this; not only as a way to thank Christine, my husband, family and friends for all their help, but as a process of accepting how my life has changed since my brain hemorrhage. I hope this gives to you the understanding that even in the worst of circumstances we are often given certain people to help you along the way. I lost in one short day everything I had worked for. This is about the process of trying to get a part of life back. I had to learn that you don't have to be the smartest, the most talented, industrious, and strongest. It's OK to just do the best you can. This book contains my thoughts and perceptions about stroke, how it feels to have a stroke, how it takes from you but also how it can give back to you. I hope that this will let you feel, understand, cherish, love and give hope to all survivors.

Foreword

Not all people have the ability to look at death, embrace it and let it change them to something better. I lost in one day all those things I felt were important. It took time, energy and consistency to fight for a new life that could give more than the pervious.

It was not until I had started to learn that I noticed those who survive trauma are those that can smile in all the bad. I want you to feel the warmth, sadness, pain and strength that I feel since my stroke. I want to offer some understanding and hope to those who can't understand and to those who do understand but don't find the strength to change the bad into good. Even in stroke we must embrace a chance to learn about others and ourselves. No one can promise that it will all come back for that is not realistic but what can be promised is that if you learn you will gain strength and understanding which then allows you to make a good life after stroke.

Who should read this book?

- ♦ All who wish to say, "I understand".
- ♦ All who wish to grow in compassion.
- ♦ All who fight to get a previous life back.
- ♦ All who want to feel stroke without having one.
- ♦ All who search for kindness.
- ♦ All who want to share a memory.
- ♦ All who want to "see" but can't.
- ♦ All who want to find compassion.

Author's Note

Some of the names in this book have been changed to protect the privacy of others. This book was developed from my viewpoint on how I felt during the time periods portrayed. The purpose of this book is to share my thoughts and views as I saw them. The book is only a recollection of how I felt as I struggled to make some sense of the stroke and what it did to me.

Chapter 1: The Stroke

The first day

I remember having the stroke. I remember the incredible pain in my head and others weeping around me. What sticks out in my memory is when I try to recall the weeks of life I lost when I couldn't physically see or intellectually feel. I guess if I was to start at the beginning, it would have to be the day I had the stroke. The day was February 21, 1997. My friend Chris had come to visit and we had a lot of fun talking and playing gently with our children. Chris took a picture of Alexa (my newborn) and I before she left. That single picture would become the lasting momento that I have of the former me. I now feel blessed for I have been allowed to live two fulfilling and distinct, but welded lives. I have been allowed to see and feel more than most. I have been allowed to strive for a spiritual self that I may not have ever had if I did not have a stroke.

It was 9PM when it started. It was as though my head had collided with a Mac truck. The pain was so intense that it paralyzed my system into a state of rocking back and forth over and over. As my fingers clenched by hair my brain drifted back and forth in a sea of nausea. I tried to remain calm but couldn't. I kept trying to tell myself that I had been through so many tests for this pregnancy that there couldn't be anything wrong. I kept trying to convince myself that it was just a really bad headache. My vision started to go. I decided to take a shower hoping that it would soothe the pain in my head. It was no more than a minute or two when I yelled to Mike, "Something is wrong!" My head was bursting into flames. My eyes felt like they were bulging out of their sockets. "I can't see!" Oh my God, Mike, Mike, something is wrong," I yelled. I could feel it. Something was terribly wrong inside of me. I could barely lift my drenched body onto the bed. He called the Doctor. He called my mom to come and watch the kids. I yelled and screamed; "I can't wait! Take me now! Get the neighbor to watch the kids!" Our neighbor came over and Mike held me as he led me to the car. It was night but even the faint light from the moon reaching between the clouds of rain hurt my eyes and my head. So with a blanket over my head we rushed to the hospital.

It was that first night that the stroke started to take from me. It took my sight, my brain, my self-confidence and my person. It took the pure sense of who I thought I was. I did not realize that I had lost some of these things permanently until much later. I would later be admitted to the intensive care unit for a brain bleed. I have often asked myself why my life was spared. Why didn't I die? It took me a long time to understand that it was because I was to learn from all of this. I was destined to learn and to speak of what had happened to me. I am to help teach all those I can about stroke. I am to help those who haven't gotten their speech back, who haven't gotten enough sight back to drive, who haven't gotten some ability to read back, who haven't gotten some ability to write back, who haven't gotten some ability to remember back, and for those who haven't gotten a life back that they should feel proud for surviving.

My hospital stay:

We all have memories when it comes to being in the hospital or visiting someone in the hospital. I myself have been hospitalized several times for both major and minor problems but none of those stays are like this one. The shame and embarrassment I felt each day when they would roll me over, bathe me and shoot me full of morphine would have a long-lasting effect on me and how I perceive the medical community as a whole. When you have just given birth and are still healing to have a male nurse bathe you is catastrophic mentally. Combine the inability to comprehend the stroke and its damage to the brain with the effects of having a child at home while people poke and prod you as though your not there is humiliating and depressing to say the least. The inability to express my concerns, wishes and embarrassment would cause nightmares for months. My mind had already been raped of its ability to communicate successfully. That was very obvious in my conversations. To then feel that my body, the only one I have was being used, poked, prodded and cleaned without my understanding was damaging. It was so damaging that I could not even tell my husband about how hurt I felt during that hospital stay. I could hear them talking about me in the halls. They talked <u>about</u> me but not <u>to</u> me. It was only Doug, a male nurse who didn't bathe me, who talked to me. He tried to help me understand what was happening. Even though I didn't really understand then, I remember his gentle hand on mine as he tried to comfort me when the pain was so unbearable.

Doug was not there the day the man bathed me. I think he would have stopped it. I think he could have sensed my embarrassment. Even though I am not the conscious self I was, the fact remains that I still feel. Just because a nurse or a doctor seems to has no sense of feeling for the physical self of a patient you must understand that I am still a human being with a heart, a soul, feelings and passions. The medical community is trained to disconnect themselves from their patient as a person. That is both good and bad. It is good that they look directly at the physical problems at hand but it is also bad that I know my body and me better than anyone and that should always be considered. When I realized that there are both good and bad doctors I learned that I have to take the steps and measures to make sure that I know the difference between the good ones and bad ones. It is not enough just to trust the medical license of the physician or surgeon, for just like a used car there are lemons. I have learned that I prefer to have physicians that treat me with a bed side manner that tells me that they care about what I think and feel.

I have learned that tests may be painful and seem cruel at times but are often necessary to help us physically survive. We must learn that each painful test has a purpose and that it strengthens our ability to survive. We survived the worst when we had the stroke now we must learn from it. The tests and recovery should be treated as a reaffirmation of our strength of will, spirit and soul. So when all feels lost and you have been torn down remember that your inner strength is something that no one can take from you.

The Priest

Now I have always been a spiritual person and a firm believer in God. I would soon learn that my beliefs would be tested again and again. When the Priest came in and gave to me my "last rights" it was then that I started to realize that I was REALLY sick. I really had no perception of how bad off I was until then. I know they kept giving me shots of morphine to deaden the head pain but because I still dreamt of my children, job and life I had no real perception of being asleep almost all the time. I also had no understanding or perception that they were only dreams now. Dreams of a past life that I would struggle with for a very long time. My waking hours were far and few between. When I spoke I couldn't understand why they looked at me funny. I would realize later that my speech had been affected by the stroke but today I do not understand.

I don't know what time it was, nor do I know if it was day or night, I don't know if it was a rainy, snowy or a sunny day. What I do know is that it was at this instance, this moment in time, I knew that death was upon me. That it

When I Learn . . .Surviving Stroke with Pride

was not a figure I could not see nor a voice I could not hear but it was I.

As I lay there trying to forget the pain in my head the quiet soft hand of my husband took my right hand. There was an eerie silence a dark lonely still in the air. It was only interrupted by a unfamiliar voice. It called my name and asked me to pray. It spoke so loudly that it seemed to pierce my ears. The priest recited "bless…..her…lord…watch over…her…to live with you…that she will find her way." I held his hand as tight as I could, I thought my fingers would break. I fought the tears that were streaming down my face from my heart. My silent plea was that I would not go now. I kept thinking "Please dear God, not until they are grown."

He said, "Donna do you believe?" "Yes", I said then he sprinkled the holy water and made the sign of the cross on my forehead. I could barely make out his face. He was gray and in tears. It was that single tear, as I clenched his hand, that told me it was almost time, almost time to die. I wasn't really afraid because of the pain. The pain made me want an end, almost welcome it. I didn't think I would die until then. Until his cross, his bright glistening cross-shimmered in front of me. Is this all there is? Where are the lights? Where is heaven? The pain is still here so I must still be alive. We said "Amen" and I fought to release his hand. I could hear Mike's tears, I could feel his fear, and I can see his heart is drenched with sadness.

God, I had this baby, I gave her life like you wanted me to. Why do you want to take mine now after all of this? I need time; time to help her grow to finish the job you gave me and to make sure that her life is not measured by my own. The still of time, as it sat there not knowing if it was to keep ticking for me, was unbearable. My chest hurt, my heart hurts, my heartburn's and now my soul hurts too. The painful realization that life's precious breath, precious memories and kiss from your child can be lost in a second was killing me. It did not take but the voice of a priest to tell me that God may be coming. Coming for me.

As I hear the nurses wrestling around and couldn't hear Mike, I wondered if I would wake up. I thought this must surely be a dream. I can not die now, not after all of this. He placed his hand on my shoulder and I awoke. I dozed off again from my dreams. He confirmed it was not a dream the priest had come. Who asked for him? They think I will die? That damn Doctor! Why wouldn't he listen to Mike? I shouldn't be laying here like this. I should be at home with my children. Why? Who gives you the power to tell me when to live and when to die, who gave you the right to say my life was not worth your time, time that you are paid and were paid for.

They poked me again and I fell fast asleep reliving my life in my dreams. I kept asking what was happening and why I am so very tired? The words I could say, "I had a stroke" that's what they said. "I had a stroke but I can't see." Just let me sleep. When I sleep there is no pain. I am not afraid to die. I am beginning to crave it and praying for a moment of no pain and peace. Peace and solitude, that is what I need now. Death awaits me and I am ready. "Dear God help Mike raise our children to know that I love them." I was asleep again.

When I woke back up I heard Mike's voice telling me that Karen was there. She moved to my left and I peered as hard as I could to see her. I held their hands and told them "I love you both very much." "I at this moment have the two people who mean the most to me with me." At that second, for that precious second, I felt no pain only the love and energy they were wishing for me. I was asleep again. How come I keep waking up? I still don't understand. "It's OK Lord you can take me now, I am at peace." He didn't take me and I still don't know why.

The Test

My nurse came to me he whispered to me Donna we have to run some tests. They told me my brain was bleeding. I had a stroke. How could my brain bleed? I was hurt in the head? What does that mean my brain is bleeding? How can you tell my brain is bleeding? Doug answer me! Why won't he answer me? Doug please help me! How can my brain bleed? Like a bloody nose? He looked at me. Donna it's all right. Can't you hear me? Can't he understand what I am saying? Why won't he answer my question?

First they make me put my head, my hurting head; boy does my head hurt, on this rock hard towel. Why does my brain hurt so badly? Donna they are going to put the pins in your head to measure the electronic pulse of your brain activity. I screamed, "What the hell do you mean your going to put pins into my brain? Now where is Mike? Mike I need help, please help me they want to puncture my brain why do they want to do that? If they put a needle in my head it will burst. I will surely die then. Lord don't let them do this to me. My heart is racing where's Mike, Mike, Mike, Mike, Mike, I need you to stop them! Make them stop my head it hurts so badly. My neck is hurting. She keeps making me put my head on this thing and it hurts my neck. Oh now what if I get paralyzed from this? I had just had disk surgery months before I found out I was pregnant. I had just gotten out of a Philadelphia brace as the disk between C-5/C-6 had ruptured compressing my spinal cord. Emergency surgery was performed to replace the blown disk and remove it to relieve the pressure on my spinal cord. Now this lady was hurting my neck. Make them stop my head and neck is hurting so bad. She doesn't care I keep telling her but she say I have to do this. Why I didn't ask for this I didn't say I want you to stick pins in my head, hurt my brain, and my neck. Doug I need a shot. He said, Donna we can't give you pain medication until after all the tests are finished. They won't come out right. I don't give a shit if they don't come out right. Why are they killing me? Do they want me to die? Did I hurt them somehow? What did I do? What is going on? Make them tell me what is wrong with me. Donna you had a stroke. We need to see if your brain is still bleeding and see if everything is ok. Is this ok Doug? Do they have to do this? Yes Donna. Ok you promise it's needed. Yes. Ok I trust you.

I held my head on that rock hard towel for an eternity. She's just taking her time. Look at her holding a grand old conversation while I die her in pain. Maybe she likes this making pain. Doug please where are you? You can make her stop. Close your eyes Donna. My eye's aren't open what do you mean close them? I am afraid I don't understand this. I'm fine. I am just tired. If you let me rest like all the other moms I will be fine. I'm done Donna. "I hope you get better," she said. My head is swimming in circles.

Who's this? Who are they? Donna the ambulance drivers are here. Don't worry I'm going with you on this one. Doug where are they taking me? They have to take pictures of your brain. You have to stay still. I'll be there Donna don't worry, I'm not leaving you. His voice was a source of comfort in all this confusion. Doug would never make or let them hurt me. I relaxed until we reached the door to the Cat Scan machine. God my head hurts make it stop. Make the pain go away. Doug may head my head please make it stop. Donna take a deep breath I will give you pain medication when we get back to your room. A voice say's OK Mrs. Brady are you ready? Am I ready? What kind of question is that? Do I have a choice? Has any one person asked me how I feel about all of this? You tell me you seem to have all the answers. OK Mrs. Brady we are going to strap you down. You have to stay still, if you don't we have to repeat the tests. You will have three tests it will take 1 ½ hours.

When I Learn . . .Surviving Stroke with Pride

After the first test I was ready to get out of the hole that put me in. Why are they shooting at me? Kill me now. Are you just trying to tease me? The machine gun goes boom boom boom, tick tick tick tick really fast so fast it makes me nauseated. Bam bam bam like a jackhammer as it pierces each particle of my being. God I am going to die right here in this machine. Let me die or get me out of here. Right now! It hurts! It hurts! Make it stop. Make it stop hurting so much. I think I passed out because they said, "Ok your finished wait here," like I was going to just get up from all these straps and walk away. I was in a gown with my rear hanging out. Maybe you should be the one lying her. Mrs. Brady we have to repeat part of the test. Why? I stayed still just like you said, I was in tears. I stared crying I can't do this anymore. Why won't they listen? It would be much later that I realized my speech was not my words. What my brain was saying was not what my mouth would sound.

So what seemed like a day in the torture chamber with the enemy ripping each thread of my life, Doug got me back to my room. He told them, "Drive you have better get her back fast." She can't take much more.

Donna we're back. Here's your painkiller you sleep now. Get some rest. Where's Mike? He'll be back. Remember he went to get April from school. Oh ok April. I miss her. I was out again for how long I don't really know. I woke with my mom standing there very quietly and not saying a word. Hi muuooomm, I mumbled. Hi honey how are you feeling? OK. That's all I could muster before I was out again.

My day or nights or day or night what ever it was would haunt me for months. The feeling of helplessness, the realization I was dying and the will to die wouldn't just go away over night. I would learn that I had to work for life and learn to love life again, maybe tomorrow. They will let me go home tomorrow. I was fast asleep again.

Donna Brady

The hospital therapist

I don't know her name nor who sent her. She came in and gave me a pad of paper and a pencil. There was a calendar on the wall next to the television. It was high up to my right side. My vision loss is on the right side so when she seated herself to my right I had to turn my head around to see her. I don't remember much about her looks just that she had a white coat on. I couldn't read the tag but I thought it was due to my bad vision.

She introduced herself and I believe she shook my hand, although I can't remember for sure. She asked me questions about why I was in the hospital. I repeated those things I had been told. "I had a stroke," I said. I believe I gave her the correct answers. To this day I do not know if I did or not.

She then pointed to the sheet of paper on the wall that had black writing on it. She asked me if I could see it. I shook my head yes. I could see something there. I had to concentrate to keep my eyes from wondering. It feels like they have a mind of their own. They keep wondering back into my head each time I try to think. I try not to think much because it makes my head hurt that much more. I never knew that thinking or having a thought could be so painful. It makes my head burst into a hot scorching array of pain. She said, "I want you to read it to me." I couldn't read it at all. I told her I couldn't read it but with a caveat, I don't see well you know. Legally blind is what I remember the words to be. I had no idea nor did it dawn on me until now that I just told her I could see it but couldn't read it. If I can see it I must be able to read it. She asked me, "Do you know what it is?" "Yes," I nodded. But I couldn't find the words to describe it. I could picture it in my brain but not its name. I know I know what it is. I recognized it. I tried to explain what it was but the words weren't there. I think I told her I know but can't remember the name. I'm really not sure what the words were that I used to describe the calendar. I was faintly aware that what my mind spoke my voice did not express.

She asked me to write something. I think I could spell my name well because she left me the tablet of paper and pencil. It's ironic because I really didn't know what to do with the paper and pencil after she left. She told me to "practice." I thought I was fine. What am I supposing to "practice?" I can't see that well that's it. I did not fully understand what that single comment would mean to me or my life. I had no inkling that my life had changed forever. Practice. "Practice what?" I kept asking myself. Did she give me something to do? She wrote some things on my thing that hung off of the wall by the door. You know why they put your charts on the wall? They know when you're as sick as I was that you couldn't get to them. They were the only ones that knew I wouldn't be able to read it. I often wonder, if I had the strength, energy and fortitude to get to that chart, when I looked at the writing, would I have realized I couldn't read, or would I blame it on the doctor's bad penmanship? Bad penmanship I am sure. It is hard to recognize and understand the problem at first. I felt normal inside. How can I feel so normal but be so abnormal? This is one of the problems with brain injury. You feel normal inside even though the outside isn't normal anymore. My brain had been injured and it would take weeks and months to realize that I was not the same. It would take months of therapy before I genuinely understood what had happened to me.

Two weeks later

Now I really don't remember many specifics about what happened the weeks immediately following my stoke but what I do know is that my family and friends were there in both spirit and concern. The hospital stay was filled with anxiety of not really knowing what had happened. I couldn't see well and couldn't eat much because eating caused my head to hurt. I thought my inability to reason, remember, and read would return when my vision did. Doctors came in and out. Lots of shots, noise and lights that hurt. I was in a total state of confusion and misunderstanding of what I was really getting ready to embark on. I remember being able to repeat the words, "I had a stroke." I had no real understanding of what that meant. I was able to mimic those around me pretty well however left on my own I could not get though the simplest of tasks. To repeat the words of the nurses and doctors took all the energy I had saved from one nap to another. Trying to remember their names and faces was impossible at that time. I don't remember to this day how I got from the ER to the intensive care unit and home, nor do I wish to. I believe that is how we protect ourselves from pain. It's like the victim of a car accident that can only remember the events leading up to the accident but not the accident itself. Problem with stroke is that as your brain heals those memories start to come back but not in any real order. What may have happened first may be remember second. I can only explain it like this. Imagine that it has rained on the sidewalk pavement. The pavement regains its tan color as each individual drop of rain evaporates. The drops do not evaporate all at once or in a pattern from the outside in or the inside out. They evaporate individually. As each drop evaporates what's left is a changing splotchy patter of color until all have evaporated. A stroke is like that pavement. Your brain heals in blotchy patterns and until it is completely healed you can't fully understand what you have left.

    I started remembering things during the weeks following my stroke. I took my memories as gospel until I learned that my memories can no longer be counted on. A memory is only as good as the brain that houses it and mine had been injured. I have learned that with time the brain trust, as I call it, gets better but there is always a certain amount of doubt. Pen and paper have become my remembering tools when my brain seems to fail. The stroke has forced me to be organized and has therefore made me more efficient in some manners. For in all bad things come some good. I now have an appreciation for those who have always written their memories on paper.

Home at last

I think I remember the car ride home just because it was sunny and it really hurt my head. Light was painful. How could something that has brought me so much pleasure bring so much pain now? That would get better although it would take a very long time. Things were much different now and I would have to learn those differences and adjust to them.

When my children entered the door I remember how hard they hugging me. I also remember not wanting anyone to touch me because of the head pain, it hurt so badly. Each place on my body felt the pain in my head. I could not escape it. At times it was so unbearable that I would pass out from the pain only to realize that the only time I was not in pain was when I was asleep. The girls were good they tried to be so quiet and helpful. I yearned to run and play with them even though I knew I couldn't. I would ask them a question and they would ask me to repeat it. I was learning that sometimes my words were really mixed up but I didn't know how to make the words come out right. I still blamed this on my vision. Most times I had to be told that the words did not make sense. I don't know how long it was before I started therapy or what the term "therapy" really meant. Mike told me later that I started that very next week. When Mike told me that I was going to go to therapy I really thought that meant I was crazy. We are not socialized to understand that "therapy" means many good things. To me it would soon mean to learn how to cope. At that moment, I could only envision the white coats, windows with bars on them, and padded walls. Mike loaded me, the kids, and my sunglasses into our SUV. My leather coat would replace the glasses before we even got out of the driveway because the bright sun felt like searing pokers to my brain.

We finally arrived at the hospital. This was the fist time I remember using valet parking. I wanted to walk on my own but had to use a wheel chair. I was very angry with Mike for making me use a wheel chair. I am strong. I am an athlete my body has never failed me. He had to remind me that I don't even have enough strength to walk to the bathroom on my own. He was right, there was no way I could manage the stairs, the elevator and the offices. The vision I had of the wheel chair depressed me. That was when I started to realize how weak I was. Mike put Alexa in my lap, which terrified me because I was so afraid I would drop her. I was not afraid because of my lack of strength but because of my vision. I thought all my problems were as a result of my inability to see well. I held on to my soft baby girl so tight that I am surprised I didn't' break her. Mike pushed me through the door of a place that would become my home. This would be the place where I would begin to learn about the new me. It would be here that I would not worry about whether they understood or not because they did. This is the place that would only know me for who I am now, not who I was a short three weeks ago.

Chapter 2: Therapy

The first day of therapy

I remember learning as a young child that things are not always as they seem. That in life we will encounter those that we do not understand. Those that we can not fully appreciate until we ourselves have learned. I met this lady my first day in therapy, her husband had a stroke about a month before me. He had both cognitive and physical difficulties from his stroke. He looked just like me. He was in a wheel chair too. I kept thinking he is just like me why would she say these things. I recall she kept telling me how lucky I was to be so young and have a stroke. Now for someone who had her stroke six days after the birth of a child, had limited vision, whose speech was not normal, who would soon learn that she couldn't read or write, I was not feeling as lucky as this lady kept tell me I was. It hurt to listen to her words and I resented her for saying them. What is amazing is that on that particular day I really had no perception of what and how the stroke had affected me. That my life, my thoughts and my perceptions had already changed. I would soon learn of those changes. I would soon begin the process of accepting and working on the new me. I would meet this lady two years later. I would not remember her until she told the story of her husband. He still has speech and physical problems. This encounter would be after my therapy was over. After I was back working. After I had learned to accept the deficits that remained. After I had taken all that bad and turned into something good. It would be then that I would learn that she saw in me something that her husband didn't have that day, faith, hope and spirit. I could still smile and he couldn't. So now I do not resent her for what she said because I know that it was because she herself was hurting over what she saw in me when compared to her husband. So this is how I learn now each moment of the day, each second of my life, and each breadth that I take.

The day my real learning began

"Hello, I am Christine," she said or at least that's what I remember. I can distinctly recall that she had a white coat on and a pen in her left hand. She shook Mike's hand; she wore black shoes, and seems very tall to me. Pretty funny how everyone seems tall when you are in a wheelchair. What was her name again? I could not remember what she said nor did I really care at that point. I am fine I just can't see that is all that is wrong with me. It would not be until I received the cognitive skills test results that I would realize the impact of the stroke and even then I would not full understand. When the brain has been injured it takes time to learn. Things that were instant are now taking hours, days and weeks to recognize. The process to relearn is long, frustrating, and difficult but is also very rewarding. One thing for sure, you may want recovery for me but it is up to me to want it bad enough to work for it. Now when I learn it is embedded into my heart and my spirit. My sight is not only the process of my vision but of my heart and soul. When I "see" I can remember and feel. When I feel I know I am alive.

I don't know what day it was but I do remember it was a Friday because I was so depressed after this session that I wanted, wished and prayed that I would die. I did not want to live anymore. How could I possibly get back to where I was? As Christine read the test results to me I started to realize with each word that my eyes were not the cause of my problems. My eyes were merely a tool that let me see the letter, and to focus with. I could not read anymore, I could not speak well, I could not remember, I could not write, I could not do ANYTHING! I stared at the wall

When I Learn . . .Surviving Stroke with Pride

trying not to let her into the pain I was feeling. What has happened to me? Why? Why now? Why me? I don't understand. The sheer realization that the physical healing of my brain would not give me back my life was staring at me. I thought I had already started working on recovery but I had barely begun. On this particular day I resent everything and everyone that touched my life. I hated God for letting this happen. I resented her for telling me these things. That is when my healing really started. That is when the spirit of life and love starts to try and creep back into the empty space of my heart and soul. So now I know that learning in not always easy. It is not as easy as it use to be. I could not just rely on remembering for that could be taken away in a moment of pain.

I asked Christine if anyone gets it all back. She asked me if I really wanted the answer to that question. I told her yes. I had to know. I pushed her for information. A part of me needed the hard cold facts no matter how painful those facts may be. I asked her again and she finally said, "Some do but most don't fully recover." Oh my God! I was screaming inside and did not know where or who to turn to. What do you mean? With the tears filling my eyes and my chest searching for comfort, I kept telling myself I can't do this! I can't take this! You are lying to me. You have to be lying to me. How could I lose all I have worked for in a few weeks? No, I don't believe it! I wouldn't believe it until later. I didn't realize it until later. I didn't learn that day. That day I fought to keep learning away. I didn't want to learn, and I wouldn't let myself believe, because if I rejected all she was saying then I could deny it. If I didn't face it then it wasn't possible and it wasn't real. If I didn't see it, then it wasn't true. There are times when we must learn through sadness and in despair for this enables us to turn it back into hope, promise and peace. For once we have had peace in our lives we can always, with work, find our way back to peace.

I went though my sessions doing all that was asked of me. At some point I decided that since I couldn't really kill myself I would try to get as much back as fast as I could. I will prove them all wrong, so I thought. Once I decided that healing was better than death I focused on healing, on learning, on both physical and mental strength, on hope and on proving my life was worthy of respect. One thing that stroke takes from you that people don't often want to admit or talk about, is you self worth. It deprives you of your confidence. It makes you a child. It makes you depend on others who use to depend on you. It takes all of your dignity. It takes in one short moment all you have worked for your whole life. It says to you, "I will not give it back unless YOU and only YOU work at it each day, with all your heart, all your soul, and all of what remains, and even then, I will not promise you the world." I did try to hurt myself once. I remember that day. Mike and I had a disagreement over something that I thought I had done but hadn't because I frankly didn't remember not doing it. It was that realization that I had no control over my thoughts and my learning that led me to hitting my head against the wall, as hard as I could, hoping that one blow would take the rest from me including my life. It was not to be. That set me back a bit in therapy but farther ahead in my will to get better. We must all sacrifice at times to learn. These sacrifices provide the sight we need to fully understand our potential. Months later I would tell her what I did and be surprised by the reaction. The day I told her we both learned. I learned that I could not expect anyone to fully understand how I felt because they are not I. She learned that even those that seem to be doing so well can often hide behind the blank stares of understanding. It would be the understanding that we both learned that would further the bond of friendship we could share.

Stroke takes a mental toll, one that is not often apparent to the survivor. I would not face the trauma mentally for months to come. I only focused on learning. Learning was the one thing that I could focus on. It would be the only thing for months. I had no perception of time anymore so the length of time it took to learn was very inconsequential to me. It may have hurt those around me to see how slow my improvements and reasoning were but for me I had no concept of speed. My mind would race a million miles an hour even though my ability to express it would be at a snails pace.

I remember trying to hide my problems from anyone that touched me. If I could pretend that I had not changed it would come true. If I could make myself forget what it has done to me I could just ignore it. That may get you through the darkest days of desperation but it does not provide healing and acceptance. We all heal in different ways, in different manners, and at different speeds but we all must heal. We all must face the changes. We must accept them and come to terms with them and their impact in our lives. It is when we finally realize that the process of healing is a life long task that we are set free from the mental burden of stroke. It was when I was set free from the embarrassment of my deficits that I realized that I had a purpose. That I had been given a gift of survival, that I had been touched with the presence of faith. That I understood and was given the precious insight to life before my physical death, I was allowed to see when others can't until it's to late.

My first big assignment

I wrote the following pages near the end of my speech and language therapy. I had wanted to show myself, Christine and the world just how far I had come from the first day I entered her office. I wanted to give her something back for all that she had given to me. I needed her to understand just how much she had helped me so that she would never forget her importance in my life, and the life of other stoke victims. Christine did not give this assignment to me; I gave it to myself. This would be the fist time I would start writing and seem to enjoy sharing this event in my life. It would start a healing process for me. Christine knew that it would help me heal but sometimes we have to learn that on our own. Ownership of life is a very hard concept after stroke because we have learned that it can be grabbed from us instantly and without warning.

It happened to me

What's it like? You look great! Why did it happen? These are the questions and thoughts of people I have seen lately.

It's a living hell. Imagine your under water and no matter how hard you paddle and kick, you can't get to the top. The top is there, right there, you can see it, and feel it, but you can't reach it. Your brain is like the water that surrounds you, you know the word, you can taste it, feel it, but you don't know what it is called.

Now I know what friends and family really mean. I KNOW the word, you know it's not an apple or an orange, it's sour, but can be sweet. It's pink or white, my kids like it. Please! I'm hungry but I can't tell you the word. We play charades again, and again, and again, but I still crave the fruit. Yes, it's a fruit, but I can't remember the word. What is it called? I know it's there, I can hear it, why can't I say it. It's not fair!! Why ME!!

Haven't I been through enough? He responds, "Yes honey, a grapefruit, is that what you want?" "Yes, thank you." "I will get it for you." Thinking it's two hours later I eat the grapefruit and complain about how long it took him to give it to me. In reality it was a few minutes. I have no perception of time, night, or day anymore. This I will have to work on for what seems an eternity. Time, what is time and where does it go? Why is this so hard? I don't understand what has happened to me. What was it's name? Make me remember, please Lord, or I will lose my mind. As he hands me the grapefruit I ask once again, "What's it called?". Again you tell me and never raise your voice. You are a loving man. I am lucky.

Now it's time to bathe. I hate it now, I use to love long hot steaming showers. They were my peace, mine to enjoy. Now it's not so good. It hurts. It makes my head burst into pain. I guess I now know what it's like to get shot. I have to call my husband again because I need help walking. To dry myself is a task. I hate it! I feel sorry that I am this way. I have taken his life with me. He looks tired so I pray that God gives us the strength to make it.

It's mail time again and I am ready. The cards are my solace. There must be millions. Mike check the mail. It hasn't come yet Donna. Are you sure? Yes dear. Donna, their here now. Do you want me to read them now or later? Now, right now. I need these cards. Without them I will die. He slowly reads them to me. I see that they too make him feel good. As I listen, I wonder why these people are so nice to me. I never thought of myself as a well liked person. I wonder what the picture on that one looks like. I would like to see its colors and its style. I now wish that I could see. I know what the blind man hears and fears. I wonder how he keeps going. Now I treasure the seeing world. I will be better to my body when I get better. Yes, but when. If these people are going to take time to care, whether it's for a moment or an hour, I will make myself get better. He just finished today's stack of mail and for the moment I feel good.

I never realized how loud a knock at the door could be. It makes my head hurt. I feel like I am dying. I wish the explosions would stop. Make it stop, I can't take it anymore. Think of the kids, they need you, Mike needs you, Karen, Mom and Dad, they all need you. I need my pain pills now!

Donna Brady

Where are the kids, help me hold her, my newborn, I love her more than life. Lord don't take mine, not until she is old. I don't want people blaming her. I'm weak, she's only ten pounds but I can barely hold her up. She smells so good. I can hear each breath. I made the right decision and I know it now. Please God let me live, not for myself but for her. Mike had to tell me again that her name is Alexa. Not remembering my own baby's name is torture. I pray with all my might. I wonder what she looks like. I wish I could see her better.

Where are the girls? I miss them. The smallest says to me, "please read to me mommy". I say, "I can't, mommy can't read anymore". I cry and pray I'll get better. My oldest, she reads to me now. She asked me how to spell "love". I couldn't tell her because I don't remember, even though my heart is filled with love. She says, "that's OK mommy, I'll read to Amber". We'll pretend I'm you mommy. I cry again. She's too young to be a mom. I can't let her. Listening to myself, I keep saying, "I can beat this", but in my heart I'm not so sure this time. I'm afraid.

One of my bosses came to see me today. He said I sounded good. I told him I'm getting better. His visit made me feel good. I hope that I get everything back so that I don't disappoint them at work. That scares me. What will I do if I don't get better.

We talked about the cards and how much they mean to me. I'm lucky, very lucky that people do care. Why me, I don't know, but this is a great feeling. I'm going to work even harder to repay their kindness.

Mike, is the mail man here? "Not yet" he says as he smiles. I can hear the truck, please check. He checks again but it's not here yet. He promised to read the cards as soon as they arrive.

I hate this! I hate what has happened to me. My family is great. My friends, they're great too. How did I get so lucky. Even my speech therapist, she cares, I can tell. I wonder how things will look when I get my eyes back. Please Lord, give me my eyes, my voice, and my memory! My weeks are filled with depression and anger. The only thing I look forward to is visiting my speech and language therapist. I can't remember her name, so I ask Mike her name every time he wheels me through the door, and each time he tells me, "Christine". She's a good teacher and she's a kind person. I enjoy my lessons with her because it gives me something to look forward to.

Today is the day that I realized I can barely talk, can't read at all, can't write, and can't remember. As Mike wheels me in to the office for what they call therapy, I did not know that life as I knew it was over. Christine barely knows me but can tell I'm in pain. I think it hurts her to read the test results to me. It can't be easy to tell someone that they are now dysfunctional in almost everything they do. So much use to be easy, now its unbearably hard. I asked her if people get completely better. She says some people get better but most never fully recover. I wonder which one I am. My new word is "dysfunctional". I'm dysfunctional, I look at her and try not to cry. She said, "It's now that you are realizing what has happened to you". I told her I've lost everything. She reminds me about my kids and husband. I love them, but how good am I to them if I can't read, write, work, and take care of them. I don't want to be a living burden on my husband. He deserves better than that. She tells me it's OK to cry, but I don't want to cry in front of her. If I do I'll never stop, EVER. I think she likes me but then she's a nice person and I am her patient. She's more than a therapist that teaches me to read and write. She's more like a friend to me. I hope she doesn't mind.

Once again I died in my sleep and decided that I have to fight. I don't want my kids and husband to be with anyone but me. I silently tell her "thank you" for getting me back on track. I have to stay motivated, if I don't, I think I will shrivel up and die. Five more cards today. It makes me cry in joy that so many people care about me. "Thank you all." It means a lot to me. I could see part of the television today. That means my eyes are getting a little better.

I'm back at this place again they call therapy. Little did I know the person in the white coat that I can barely see would become more than just another doctor or nurse to me. She started slow, so she says. Seems really fast to me now. She knew more about what I was getting ready to go through than I did. At first I thought this was stupid. After all, I have a career. I have a bachelors degree, and I am on the last legs of my masters degree. I don't need this thing called therapy. I looked at the word that she wanted me to read. I looked and stared at it as hard as I could with the little bit of sight that remained, and said the word. Only the sound was in my brain, not in my mouth, and I really did not know the word after all. She said it was "cat" I thought it was "mountain". I realized then that I have a thousand mountains to climb now.

Just to speak was hard. Harder than I imagined it could be. I know what it feels like to be mute now. It came out either in mumbled noises or nothing at all. When a word did come out it wasn't the word I thought it was I said. I could feel and hear the words in my head. I didn't know until today that nothing was coming out. I couldn't even say the words that I was screaming in my head. "What's wrong with me". I started my battle today. Later I would appreciate Christine much more than I did today. I feel stupid in front of her even though she's there to teach me and help me get back what I have lost. All I could think about was that she can't be much older than I am.

My doctor says I will get better. I hope he's right. It worries me but I will keep fighting. My daughter reads better than me. She is only seven years old, but soon, with more of Christine's help, I will be able to read to her again.

Every session I try to see, to read, to write, and remember. Every day the fact I can't slaps me in the face. It gets harder each day my mind, voice, and sight stay empty. I'm starting to wonder if I will get better. Two weeks and I will be driving they said, three months later I finally do. I work hard on my lessons and try the best I can.

He looks exhausted and I am worried about him. He's doing so much for me, I wonder how long he can keep up this pace. We cried today. Those people at work are very giving. I hope I can tell them how much I appreciate it. They have donated a lot of sick leave to me. I am very grateful. We hugged and I cried harder. I think to myself what have I done to deserve this kindness. I pray that God blesses each one of them.

I learned how to tell time today. Little did I know it would take weeks to relearn how to do this. I feel like I'm back in first grade. I have lived one childhood already. Why must I live through another? I wonder if it was this hard the first time. Although everyone is supporting me through this, I feel degraded having to ask what it says, what's the time, and say it again because I don't understand any of it anymore.

Once I master time again, I have to learn money, how to dial the phone, and eventually make spaghettios on the stove. I feel like a small child fighting to get out of a terrible nightmare. I'm starting to realize that Christine is right, it will take time. I am also starting to realize that she may be my only way back to the real world, or at least the one I knew before this. Time that I don't have. I am watching it, it's like a old silent movie all tattered and broken. Each frame makes up a part of my life that I have lived and a part that I have yet to live. Now as each frame fades away, with it are my hopes and dreams. Maybe tomorrow will be a better day.

I received two recruits for promotion in the mail. I cried harder than I did when Walsh College sent me an application for my next class. I often don't think it's fair that life for everyone else continues while mine fades away. I hate what has happened. I asked Mike to throw these things away because their to painful to see. Guess it's a good thing that I can't read because if I could I would probably torture myself through the agony of each word.

I say to myself today, while he reads five more cards, "I am lucky." I have a good life, wonderful children, loving husband, caring family, and thoughtful friends. I am blessed. I still don't know why he still loves me. He's good to me. I don't deserve him, thank you honey, "I love you."

I'm getting better. My sister is here comforting and helping me. I love her. She has always been there for me. I have tried to tell her how much, but I always cry. She knows it, but one day I will tell her without crying. She is a good sister, the best. When she leaves I give her a hug. I struggle to let her go because I am afraid that I will never enjoy the things we use to do together. Thank goodness I still have long term memory left. Each day I relive the softball games, basketball tournaments, my awards at work, my last contract negotiation, and wonder if those are also lost forever. Memories are only good if they make you feel good when you relive them. I don't know because they are only a reminder of who I use to be a few months ago.

I went to work today right after therapy, I told Christine, "I am nervous". She knew by looking at me. As I walked out she said, "Donna, you'll be OK". Everyone tells me that, but for the first time since this all began, I believed it. Today may be the last time she teaches me and I am sad. I wrote a card for her. I hope it means to her what it means to me. My eldest daughter wrote a message to her that went something like this:

I like you because you do homework with my mommy.

I think you're beautiful because my mommy can do homework with me now.

I cried, for April is only seven and she has already learned what it is to be grateful and compassionate. Work feels good. Everyone is so kind. They tell me I look good and they are happy I am back. I tell them thank you, and some cry with me.

It's Friday, June 5, 1997. Today is a glorious day. It's been almost four months now since my struggle began. I gave Christine the card I wrote to her. She has helped me learn to accept the new me. I am glad I met her. I will never forget her. She gave me more than just teaching me the things I use to know. She listens to me and never judged my words, and some of them were really bad. Some people say, "but that's what she is paid to do." I tell them, she was paid to teach me, which she did. Her thoughtfulness and kindness she gave to me for free. Through my tears she could make me laugh and feel good. That was a hard task back then. My life seems to be getting back to some normalcy and that feels good. As I walked outside, I looked up to the sky and told my husband "I love you with all my heart and soul", my children, "I will be there for you always", my sister, "my life is not complete without you", my parents "Thank you for believing in me", to Christine, "Thank you for teaching and helping me", and God "Thank you for letting me stay a while longer". To each and everyone of you that helped me, "Thank you".

Someone asked me, "What is the worst part?" I had to think hard because it's all bad. There's not much good about it. I finally said, "It's accepting the loss. That's the hardest part." Knowing that no matter how much physical and mental healing takes place, you will never be who you knew you could have been. That's the hardest part.

The best part is that you learn what life really means. You change, you look at your priorities and the priorities of others and realize that because of this, you have learned more since this happened than most learn in a life time.

I am a strong person, I know that now. I am a caring person, I know that too. I am a changed person, that's obvious. What I do know is that if I can survive this, anyone can. If I can make it, so can you. I think a lot of people learned a little about themselves because of my misfortune.

If nothing else good came from this, it has reaffirmed my belief that people are good to one another in time of crisis. Each person I meet, I try to learn one thing from them. I met a bad doctor in this and learned that even I can hate. I've never hated anyone before. That hard. I met a great person that showed me that even a stranger can care, "Thank You Christine".

As I took a long hot shower, I thought about all I have written here. The question a co-worker asked came back into my head. What's it like? I guess I would finally say that it's like a child learning to walk for the very first time. A child grabs on to mom and dad as they learn to lift themselves up to take that first step. I used everyone to lift myself up. Like a child who selects their favorite blanket as security. Christine became that for me. I told her once that she was my stable factor. Like a child who must venture out on their own, I too had to learn to walk on my own again. Each new step was scary but now I have taken many. Like a child I will fall but like that same child, I will get back up and try again.

The day Christine received this is the day that this child walks on her own again. Only each step I take now, is a step as an adult that has learned to accept, deal with, and conquer my brain's new limitations. I see the world in a new light with a new voice and a new direction, and I am grateful.

Lost in surgery

Well I have been driving for a little while now. I don't have to look at my map anymore. What I failed to realize is that not only do I have to take the same path each day but park in the same parking space. Today for some unknown reason they closed the parking lot I usually park in. Well that wasn't so bad. I found a spot and walked to my therapy session. It was not until a gentleman stopped to ask who I was looking for when I realized I was not in the right area of the hospital. He startled me when he asked me for her name. It had taken me months to remember Christine's name without it being written on the palm of my hand. I couldn't remember it. I was panicking at the thought that I really didn't know where I was. I showed him my blue folder that has her name on it. He told me I needed to go to the other side of the hospital. I was at the main hospital not in the medical building. He told me to go back down to the first floor, take a right past the windows where the front door is, keep on that wall around the corner to the next elevator. One funny thing is how to you stop someone who is trying to help you and tell them you don't have any idea what they are telling you. Directions to me are like a foreign language you smile and nod you head but you really don't know how to get there any better than you did before. He told me I needed floor three not five. Well after my face finished cooling down from the complete and total embarrassment I walked into therapy. I did think about telling Christine what happened but couldn't, the humiliation I felt was awful. What would she think? How could I tell her that after three months of therapy three days a week that I didn't know where I was going? I laughed it off as being in nowhere land and not paying attention. I didn't tell her or anyone else until I learned that getting lost would now be a new part of my life. In my eyes I was already stupid how would that look? I would just be dumb and dumber. It could happen to anyone right?

I often thought that everyone has the same problems I do. I would finally learn that people say, "Oh I do the same thing all the time." They do this out of caring and trying to be nice. They mean no harm. Your friends and family want you to feel the way you did before, but I can't. It is unrealistic to think that you won't change after something like this. We are given signs and symptoms and it's not until we learn to accept ourselves for who we are that we finally learn that it's ok to be the new me.

Leaving Therapy

I have been in therapy for some time now. We had fought the insurance company to keep my sessions going. Every six weeks offered a new struggle. I went back and forth emotionally trying to come to terms with what felt like another loss to me. I had become very dependent on my sessions. I was worried that I would not be able to cope without Christine.'s direction.

The time was near even I could tell. My sessions were coming to an end. It's like walking through a tunnel that had started so dark and bleak. The realities of my fears were surfacing. The vast tunnel offered no light or hopes on its wall. This tunnel of learning was filled with ups and downs, with craters and low hanging ceilings. I could barely see a small faint glimmer of light that seemed to be in front of me. I don't think it was the coat she wore but the strength of her spirit that I could see. I focused on that light so hard that I didn't give any cares to the other things that surrounded me. Other problems were brushed to the side for another day.

The insurance had approved a final six sessions. Six weeks and this will end. How will I do this on my own? Who can I confide in to help me stay on tract? Mike was my emotional strength but there were things that I felt about me that I couldn't bother him with. How do I tell him I am afraid of life? He is my soul mate I would not be alive if it were not for him. Christine taught me how to function again. She gave me back that part of life that was stripped away from me like a piece of candy in a child's hand before she has eaten her dinner. I felt like a child for many of these months. I did not want it to end. I was afraid for it to end. I had come to look forward to each appointment and see and feel my progress. Now in six short weeks it would be gone, and I would be left on my own to cope with what the stroke has done to me.

Christine was up front and honest with me about my abilities and progress. I believe we were both surprised that I had come so far. A miracle I think. I look and talk with other stroke victims and I know that I am luckier than most. That I have a life back and for that I should be grateful.

It was not until that final day that the reality hit. This was it, there was no more. Christine had told me that she had done all she could for me. That now my recovery would dependent on my ability to continue using what I had learned. She told me read read read to be a better reader. "Practice is what it will take," she said. So I continue to read each day not by choice but out of the intense desire to get better, to be where I was before the stroke. It will take time for my abilities to stabilize. Only time will tell me how far I can really go. Hard work is the only way for me now. I have learned that yes I have deficits but that is ok. I can cope with what is left. I may never fully accept my deficits for that will keep me working on them but one thing I know now is that my new life is better for having learned.

Today is my last day with Christine. I remember that day so vividly in my mind. I walked in the secretary said "hello." Christine soon appeared and handed me some forms to fill out. I had to finish those before I went back to her office. As I read each word of each question all I could think was that precious minutes were ticking away. I was losing precious seconds of final recovery and time with her. It took me quite a long time to answer the questions because I read so slowly. I hate how long it takes me. I get up and hand the secretary the forms. I walk back to her office. I sat down in my chair for the last time as a patient. I was sad that it was over. The reassurance and consistency was gone.

We talked business for a while then we chatted a little. She gave me my final assignments to be completed at home and corrected by me. I would look up and see the minute's race by and wish I could break the hands of the clock. It was the same clock I had learned to tell time on again.

I began to examine the room. I tried to etch each nook and cranny into my brain. I did not want to ever forget this day. Forget all she had done and all I had accomplished here in this room. This small corner of my world would leave a lasting impression on my life. It had become a big part of me.

The clock struck 9:50AM it was time. I remember starring at it and fighting back the tears. My recovery was now over. The end of me was here. I looked at her as I slowly put my things away. I was crying inside. She stood up, that was my cue it was here, the final goodbye. I stood up and we gave each other a hug. I told her thank you for everything. She said, "I won't forget you." I had come so far from the first day when Mike wheeled me in. I said goodbye to everyone. My emotions were barely hanging on. I turned and said goodbye one last time but Christine had already started back to her office. As I pulled open the door for the last time as a patient, the tears began to flow. I now was on my own. I felt like a fledgling bird who's mom just pushed her from the nest to either save her own life in flight or fall to her death.

I walked down the hallway and stopped to look at the lake through the window. It was a sad day. I did not want to leave my sanctuary. The only place I could be and feel like the new me. I could be who I am now not who I was before the stroke. It was hard to try and make people think I had not changed, that I was still the person I use to be because I was not. The stroke had changed how I think, what I can do, how I remember and who I am. I am a more compassionate person now even more than I was before. I am more worried now than I was before. I had little control over my life and I knew that.

When the elevator opened I looked down the hallway half-wishing Christine would appear to say we made a mistake we had a few more sessions left but the elevator door opened. I walked into the elevator and said, "I will miss it here." I walked very slowly to my truck. It seemed that with each step I would glance back hoping that Christine would appear to tell me that there was more she could do for me. In my heart I knew there was nothing more she could do to help me. She had done everything, it was now up to my own brain, and my own ambition to get more back. I now had to rely on myself. Today I was forced to become an adult again. Forced to face the stroke and what it had done to me.

I find that I am more philosophical now. My mind is very complex with thoughts and feelings. The stroke has brought out a part of me that I did not know existed. I am finding that I like to write. I wrote the following and gave this to Christine. I find that I am learning things I never thought possible for someone like me. It's not all math, science and technical ability it's about spirit and the human heart. The writing is about how my mind now envisions how meeting people are not merely by chance but by grace.

A very short story, November 14, 1997

It was a dark cold winter's night when two women, who did not even know one another, were destined to meet. At the stroke of 9, the two lives started their journey. It was at the brink of death that the sprite decided to live. As the stroke touched her spirit, took her ability to reason, understand, and remember, it was the spirit of the other that would soon give back to her those things that were so quickly taken away. The spirits of the children strengthen her but the spirit of the heart helped her get through. The life of the other was also changing, although more slowly. The change would one day be understood. As she laid in the hospital bed with her brain half empty, she did not realize that it would be a new face and heart that would give her the ability to once again chase the spirit of her children.

It was a bright crisp windy day when these their lives would cross. As she was wheeled into the room, she tried to focus on what it was that she was there for. She did not really know what had happened to her. She could hear a soft concerning voice speaking to her. As she started slowly lifting her head, she focused on the white coat that seemed to be so very far away. She looked up at the woman that stood there with her bright blue eyes that seemed to somehow understand. As the soft-spoken voice asked her name, the woman in the wheelchair spoke sparely as to not give away too much, but enough to know that something was terribly wrong. As she asked herself what the purpose of this was, she concentrated on the woman, trying to focus on every word as it rolled off of her tongue. To capture each syllable, so that it could be understood, and to one day in the future, realize that what would be learned was not as it use to be.

At that moment when the first question was asked, and the first answer given, the two lives who were destined to meet crossed. With each question would come and answer, and with each answer would come understanding. It was that understanding that would take the spirit of one and allow it to fly once again. It was also that same understanding that would touch the lives of them both forever.

In the end, when two people meet and then part, the spirits are forever changed. It will be on a dark cold winter day, like the one that drove their lives to meet, that they will once again reflect on all that had happened and smile.

My way to say "thank you"

A story on saying "thank you!" It was on March 12, 1997 that a person would come into my life. She would help me regain not only my ability to read, write, remember, speak, and get thoughts, but would somehow care about me, as a person, not just a patient that comes and goes with a breeze.

It was after months of re-learning, frustration and hard work that it was coming to an end. This end would take months. The first end was in June so I gave Christine a gift to thank her for basically putting up with me and the bad things I would say. To make sure she knew and so I wouldn't forget, I wrote, "It Happened To Me." With it was a card that told her how much I appreciated what she had done for me.

The second end came a few months later, with that end I mustered up all the courage I had and walked into the Col.'s office and explained to him that therapy was ending and I wanted to give to her an award, his award for outstanding service. He looked at me, reached into his brief case, and said he would be happy to have me give it to her. This meant a lot to me, as I have not even earned that award yet. So with that metal I gave her another way of saying "thank you." Now I had already given her two things, one was from my heart and my new found ability to write again, the second was from my work because I never thought I would ever work again in any capacity.

The insurance took some time and I had a lag between my sessions but finally they returned our calls with another approval of 6 more sessions. This would be it as there was no more insurance coverage and I could not afford it otherwise. Not only did I have to go to work so that I would still improve but I had to go to help support our family. I went back to work early before I was really ready. Christine helped me try to organize my life and work so that I could cope. She helped me come up with strategies that I would find invaluable.

It was here the final and last session. I was very sad and upset. Christine was my only connection to life after stroke. She was the only person I could talk to about what was going on with the "new me." The only one that could somehow understand without having been though it herself. Christine always made me feel better. My mom had told me about a song that she loved and thought of when I became ill. It was Alabama's "<u>Angels Among Us</u>." I listed to that song and a verse that went something like "I believe there are angels among use, sent down to us from somewhere up above, to help us in our time of need, it's funny how,…someone give use a single ray of hope." I don't remember the words exactly but it was the feeling that it gave me when I heard it that I remember most. I saw Christine's face as the angel that helped me find my way. My mom sews great quilts. Some time ago, I remember Christine and I having a conversation about quilts. I remembered her saying she liked them. I asked my mom if she could make a quilted wall hanging for her. My Mom agreed that it would be a kind gesture. With that my mom made a "Angel" quilted wall hanging. On the back of the quilt I put a verse of the song and told her she was my angel. I included in the wrapped box a cassette tape of it for her to listen too. That box contained my final "thank you" to her.

I knew that Christine would give me a hard time about giving her another gift but I did it as much for me as much as I did it for her. At the close of that session I brought out the box. She started to say something to the effect of "you

When I Learn . . .Surviving Stroke with Pride

have done enough already." I said, "No, let me tell you a story." When I was 16 years old. I played basketball on the varsity team in high school. I had a friend; she was a great person. She came from a not so fortunate home where she helped take care of her siblings, five I think. Her dad was gone a lot for his job. Her mom had to work a lot of hours too. She had the job of helping care for her younger siblings after school before her parents got home. It was a very small town and no one had much so we all made due with what we had. One of her sisters has downs syndrome or some kind of problem that makes her slow, so as you may guess life was not easy for her. Terry always helped her parents with her siblings. She helped them with their homework and was basically helping fill in when her parents were at work. Terry never complained about anything. She never said a word of anger or resentment over having what seemed to be so little time for herself. I don't think I ever heard her say a bad word about anyone or anything. Terry loved basketball she joined the junior varsity team at our high school. She was not very athletic but it was something that she did for herself, the only thing that I really remember. I was not her best friend but one thing I know about her is that she had a heart of gold. Terry wanted to make the varsity basketball team, that was what she wanted more than anything. Basketball was her passion. It made her feel great. I offered to help her learn the game and the moves so that she could play better. We practiced everyday before and after school as much as she could. I taught her everything I knew about the game. I showed her every move and every corner that I had learned. She worked hard. She gave it her all everyday. Terry was a coach's dream because no matter what the circumstance she gave 110% each time. My coach asked me what I was doing I told her she wants to play on the varsity someday and I am helping her. I asked coach if she would let her sit the bench for just one varsity game. I was promptly reminded that we can only carry five on the bench and it's the end of the season. Maybe next year, she said. I was very disappointed that Terry had worked so hard and would have to wait another year to see if she would get her turn on the varsity squad. Well coach surprised me. The first game of our division series was that night. Terry ran up to me that day is school. She was so excited that she could hardly keep still, "DJ, DJ, oh my, I can't believe it, I get to sit the varsity bench tonight!!" She was smiling from ear to ear you could see it in her excitement in her eyes. She talked about it all day. It was funny because it was like she had won a million dollars! It was a great feeling to see someone so deserving of something good so happy. No matter if we won or lost it was going to be a good game. I smiled all day feeling her excitement made all the hours of practice worth it. I told coach, "thank you" and she just said, "remember she won't play just sit the bench." I told her that was OK, then coach said, "you both deserve it, you've worked hard." Well we got to the game that night and we were both hyped up. Terry was beaming as we sat on the bleachers waiting for our game to start. She was so excited that her legs were battering up and down and left to right. She could hardly control the energy that was exploding inside of her. Terry said "I am so excited!" "I know I won't play but just sitting there and giving you guys your water bottles is great!" I think about it now how that was all she needed to be happy right then. To have something good happen to her. Well as we were sitting there she started getting a headache. I thought it was just from the excitement that had been building all day. Her sister was sitting next to her and handed her two aspirins. She leaned over to me and said "DJ, I'll be right back." I told her, "Ok, but hurry coach is going to call us down to the locker room pretty soon, I'll meet you there if she comes before you get back." With this big beaming smile that only a perfect day could make, Terry shook her head and said, "Ok, I will hurry." I was laughing as she bounced down the bleachers and ran to the hall

When I Learn . . .Surviving Stroke with Pride

towards the drinking fountain. I remember like it happened yesterday that as she pushed the hallway doors open smiled at me and gave me a thumb up. That was the last time I talked to Terry. The next time I saw her was at her funeral. She died of a massive brain aneurysm on her way to the bathroom; she never even got to take the aspirin. They didn't tell me. They told me that she wasn't feeling well and they took her home. I kept thinking, "Of all days, her day, the one where her wish would come true." We won that game. I played my heart out like I always did. No one told me she had died. They only told me that she wasn't feeling well. What I didn't know was that your brain can die but your body can live with help from machines. They knew I wouldn't play if I had known that she had been rushed to the hospital in an ambulance. They were trying to protect me.

Coach told me the next day Terry was on life support. She told me that she would be coming off of it very soon but not because she would get better. Terry was brain dead. I didn't understand what that meant because her sister would tell me that she moved her foot today. Later I would understand that when the heart is beating the person might be gone. Because of who she was and her love of life all her major organs were donated. Isn't it a miracle that someone else lives through her heart and another sees with her eyes? Those people that received her organs have life as a result of my friend's death. I hope they are taking good care of her. That was a hard concept when I was so young.

After her organs were removed the machine was turned off. I lost a friend I didn't know well enough that day. I was angry because I had not told her how much her friendship meant to me. A few days before the funeral coach pulled me aside. She wanted to give Terry her varsity letter but Coach didn't have any pins to place on it. Since I was helping her in basketball they asked me if I would give her the pins off my letter jacket. I thought it would make Terry smile.

Coach said, "I will replace yours when they come in," but that didn't matter to me. I carefully removed each pin from my varsity letter. I was so careful to make sure it didn't bend or get scratched as I gently tugged the clasp apart. I gave them to coach as the tears welled up in my eyes and my throat turned into a big knot. Terry was buried in her sweat suit, with her varsity letter, and pins lying on her chest. I know she was smiling because she also had her basketball shoes with her to take to heaven. I was teased because I cried at the funeral. For some it was just a time to get off of school. I listened to her best friend talk about her love of life and people. Our basketball team dedicated that season to her. To this day I have the new paper articles. I look at her picture when I need to remember how precious life is. We went all the way to the state that year. I know that we had a cheerleader in heaven.

After telling Christine about my friend, I handed her the box. I told her that when Terry died I promised myself that if anyone ever did something special for me, I would make sure that they knew it. Without giving me a hard time she took the box that contained the final "thank you." I keep in touch with Christine so that I can remember the strength of her spirit that allowed me to see with my spirit and my heart not just my eyes. With a smirky grin I told Christine, "When I am done you will never forget me." Conceited, as that may seem to be, I don't think she will ever forget me or at least I hope not. We can only hope to touch the life of one person in our own lifetime. I wanted to make certain that somehow I gave something back to the one that touched mine.

When I talk to Christine now, I try very hard not to talk about the stroke so much. If there is to be some type of friendship from all of this, then I can't talk to her about those things I once did. So when Christine asked me, who I talk to now? I really didn't know how to answer it. I thought about it long and hard. Christine was the only one for months. I would still be comfortable talking to her about the stroke if I had too. I don't want Christine to feel like she is in a counseling session each time she sees me. No one, not even I, like to talk to someone who complains and belly aches about his or her life all the time.

Christine knows that my life is different that it use to be so I do not need to tell her how hard I perceive things (I swear somedays I think I am just imagining all of this like a bad dream that never ends). Back to the question, whom do I talk to now? Since the therapy ended there is only one person who I can talk to besides her. She is someone I work with. That's it, no one else. Christine told me that she worries about me not having anyone to talk to. She knew that she was the only one I would confide in. There were so many things that I couldn't burden my husband with. He already had too much to deal with he didn't need more. So because of my inability to share my deepest thoughts of stroke she was the only one who I did not try to hide the face and fear of stroke from. Sometimes I still find myself wanting to go back to her. I have called her and complained about my life just to feel bad because I shouldn't burden her with my problems.

Testing a new life

I clearly remember the day I returned to work because I had a speech and language session before I went. I remember how nervous I was to face those I had known for years with the new and not so improved me. It was a very bright and sunny day. It was warm and I remember looking at the sparse amount of clouds that hovered over my head and wondering if I was really ready. Christine had done everything she could do to help me. She was a source of my stability but I was doing this one on my own. She could not be at work to help me understand and manage my life. I started working only four hours a day. That was really hard.

I was so exhausted by the time I got home that I often would fall asleep before I had even changed from my work cloths. My oldest daughter would wake me when the baby would cry. I was scared and I was panic-stricken over my inability to keep myself going. The confidence I had once known was gone. I felt panic-stricken at each turn I made and each step I took.

As I drove towards the building that I had once shared with friends I started trembling inside. I was afraid of what they would think of me now. Would I recognize them? Would they see though this barrier I was trying to develop to hide my deficits? My heart was racing, my legs were shaking, and it was all I could do to keep the tears from streaming down my face. I longed and needed the protection of my isolated house and therapy environment. I had a few panic attacks prior to this day but non-like the one I was having now.

People change in times of crisis and devastating illness. There are those who want to help you and those that treat you like the plague thinking they could get it from you. I think the most surprising is that some who helped were people who I thought didn't even like me before the stroke. Then there are those, those who were your friends that are no longer because of the illness. People can be on two extremes of each other. You don't know where you fall until you get there. I had a friend with whom I thought I was close, who turned her back on me in my greatest time of need. The scorning words and hateful comments would rip though my heart like a razor blade. I would not understand why until later. I would have to learn more about people before I could "see" why she reacted the way she did.

The art of learning has a lot to do with your willingness to look deep within your own life to find the answers that were placed there years ago. We are all born with a sense of love, morality and consciousness. It is our outside self in growing up and our experiences that take and keep us from who we were born to be. I realize now that people are afraid of illness, death, and disability. That we are taught to mistrust and be hateful to the things we do not fully understand. It is in our power and up to us as individuals to seek the reasons for our fright. It is also within our power to change. You must be willing to change and accept the responsibility of your mistakes to change your own heart. You can not make me change nor can I make you change. One thing I know for sure is that if I show my best you too will be tempted to show yours. It is when we have touched the heart of someone that change happens immediately and forever. To be an inspiration is good but to inspire is better, for those that inspire cause change. Change for the good is our life's purpose. To me change means trying to make life better for all that are affected by stroke. It is our duty to teach what we have seen and learned so that we can help others understand better and accept the things we can not change. To help others see past our brains limitations and their own. We must all understand that it takes some people a lifetime to achieve and learn what it truly means to live. We must try not to be to harsh on those who just can not see what we see, who can not feel the passion we feel, and who can not see past our limitations.

Looking at the old life

It has been about two years since my stroke. That was the single day that my life and brain changed. There are days that still seem incredibly bad to me. I would be lying if I said that it's easy to have a stroke and go on because it isn't. It's very hard to try to change the old habits and form new ones, especially when it often seems the new habits are worse than the old ones. I told a friend that the single hardest thing to learn after stroke is to learn how to trust yourself again. I have learned that I communicate better since I have had to a relearn how to express my needs and wants; however, I have also learned how to hide what really hurts me. I think that as a stroke survivor we do not want to be seen as weak because most often our bodies show our weakness. There have been days that I have wanted to throw my hands up and say, "It's not worth it anymore." "Label me as handicapped and I will cruise through life as an invalent." It didn't take more than looking at my children, friends, and family to see that our lives are worth much more than our limitations. That it is up to us to give back what we have been blessed with. I truly believe that even in stroke we are blessed. Had it not been for my stoke I would be working more and more and more and spending less and less time with my children. I would have missed out on making some GREAT friends at the hospital. I would have lost the opportunity to meet other fantastic stroke victims who have taught me more about survival than an able bodied person could. So I do believe that there is a silver lining to that darkness of stroke; however, it is up to us to find it and reap its benefits. Seek it out and then hold it in your hands with all the strength that your spirit empowers you to. People talk about moving mountains. We move mountains with each word, thought, step, and day we survive stroke. We may not see the mountain move today or even tomorrow but we have a lifetime to push each grain of sand. Isn't life at its best when we have achieved something we weren't supposing to? Some may ask, "Even if it is in small amounts when compared to our former selves?" I would say, "When I learn about who I am, what my purpose is and why I am still here, I look to that mountain and know that I have learned that we all have purpose and just like each grain of sand we all have shown how easily the mountain moves."

The first book I read

I remember how hard it was to read my first book post stroke. I use to love to read and read and read. I loved words and searching them out in my life. To understood the meaning of all things lye in the words of books and speech. I was afraid to read after the stroke because it reminds me of how much I miss the ease of it and pleasure it use to give me. I could see how long and strained it took me now. I knew just how much of the words I couldn't read more or less understand. Each day I would force myself to read thinking that one-day soon it will come back. That the more I practice the easier the words would come. Now that was true to some degree but I know now that reading would never give me the pleasure that it once did. The days of speed reading and graduate courses are over. It was a blow to not only my ego but to my spirit. I often wondered why this had happened to me. What am I too learn from my inability to read? I had no answer yet.

The day I learned was the day of the stroke group when one of the members told me "It's OK Donna I can't read at all I can only walk." Now my gut sank and I felt so extremely selfish because he had been a lawyer before his stroke. Words and their meanings were his life, his being, and his soul. He had trained years to be able to manipulate and move people with his voice and words but now he had neither. It's not like the words aren't screaming in his head for if he is like me the words never turn off. They just don't go any farther. The words they come in my head but not to my mouth. They are caught in an endless spiral of nothingness waiting to be picked up my mouth as it passes by. This day I learned that we should all appreciate what we have in this life no matter how small and insignificant society tells us it may be. His value is more than just walking everyday so that his muscles will get stronger. His value is to help change the people he meets each day. He is now a teacher of men. I now value the fact I can read and write no matter how bad it feels. I value that I can express who I am and what I think in words from my mouth. I will never express as I had at one time but that is OK for if we have learned, then we did not lose it in vain. So what did I do after I had this conversation with him? I read a book. A book that would teach me that no matter how bad my problems seem there is always someone who has it worse. He taught me that day and for that I will be forever grateful. When I learn now it is forever. It is implanted into my brain like a seed and as I nourish it with compassion it grows, and so I grow, and the more I grow, the better I am and will be.

Encounter of compassion

I can not say her name for I have not seen her in a long time but she left me with a memory. I met her on a crisp day when the sun was barely peeking through the clouds. She did not like me at first or just didn't know how to take me. I am not sure why she didn't like me. I would find a compelling compassion to help her. To make her feel like I feel now not how I felt then. She has lost a lot. Her arms and legs fail here and I can see and feel her pain. I looked down deep into her eyes and I could see the misery that was once me. My heart went to her and I prayed that she would find her way back to life. I gave her my name and number and told her that if she needed me she could call. I watched her as the stroke took her sense of trust and worth. She would grab her husband, he would hug her, and then she would cry. Stroke takes and it's hard to find your way back to life. I remember she smiled the next time and told me she was glad I was there. It made me feel good. Her kind words reminded me that I have a purpose. I must do this for her and for them. I must give back for I have been blessed with many great things.

It was a few stroke meetings later that she would stand on her own two feet for the first time in front of the stroke group. She did not stand for her husband or me, she did it for herself as it should be. I was so proud of her that day! It was an exciting time for her and our group. She put aside all her pain and stood for us all to see. To watch someone stand on her own when she had been in so much pain is an incredible feeling. She has come so far I thought as a warm feeling came over me. The tears streamed down my face in joy for what she has accomplished and for what she will accomplish in the future. I learned that day that even a smile, quick "hello" or "how are you," is all it may take to give hope and happiness. A smile may not bring a life of pleasure but it sure brings a graceful moment that may live forever. A life of pleasure is built when all the smiles of your life are combined into sunshine. I have not seen her in a while but one thing for sure is that I smile when I think of her. My heart makes me work harder when I think back to these new memories that I am forming. I have now replaced all the bad ones with all the good ones that I have made as a result of my stroke. I can now laugh at myself when I do things a bit backwards. I find joy in being with others, I find love in sharing with others, and I find peace in feeling with others.

Chapter 3: Emotional Rage

Loss

Lost Reading/July 30, 1998

Today is the day not unlike any other day. The sun is shining and the breeze is warm enough that I can roll my sleeves up and feel the sun penetrating my skin. I don't know why this day is so different than yesterday or why it couldn't occur tomorrow.

The headache started days ago the steadiness of the knife jabbing into my brain is wearing me down. I know that the brain pain will eventually subside but it is now day 4 and I am beginning to worry. I can't have another stroke. If I do I want to die. This pain is making me realize that there may never be an end to my agony.

I am reading or trying to I should say a book written by a brain injury survivor. It was today that my reality really started to hit again. I picked up the book and learned that I can't read today. The simple words, the ones I learned months ago have taken a detour to another part of my brain that I can't find. My inability to remember and read haunts me today. My chest is feeling heavy. It's like when you're told that someone you care for has been injured and may not live. I want to read this book; it is starting to give me some thoughts on those situations I can't seem to explain very well.

I should feel fortunate that my short-term memory is not as bad as hers is but today my memories are almost all bad. I have not one smile to give today. She used a analogy of walking in a fog, for me it's like a bird who sees freedom and starts to fly as fast as she can to suddenly slam her face into the crisp clear window. When the window hits it is then that you are reminded that freedom from this prison called a brain is no longer an option. For with the brain there is no release for good behavior. It is like being on death row, only you didn't kill anyone nor do anything to be put there. Just lucky, I guess.

I must stop living in a world where I hope and dream for a full recovery. It is becoming very apparent that I will NEVER have my self-back. Now I must work on trying to like the self that has taken over but I realize that I don't know how. One thing they don't do with stroke is give you a help file that points to the way out. So today I pray that tomorrow I will be able to read again so I can try to learn and remember what I have read.

My greatest fear is forgetting my kids. I forget my keys; I forget my books and my purse. I often check things 3-4 times even though I know I checked, but can't clearly remember if I really did. I know and feel the author's confusion: being lost inside yourself and not realizing it until you're past your turn. Reality sets in. There is no more. I can only go down from here.

Passion

As I sit here and listen, the priest speaks of passion and having passion in one's life. He reflects back on his own passions as a young man. His passion was for politics and helping others. He speaks of how passions change as we change during our life. It can only make me wonder if he would change his speech if he had been talking as a stroke survivor.

The stroke cut short my passions as a young adult paving my way through life. I thought about my passion as a child growing up in many different states. My passion was to make friends and keep them, for I hated saying good-by. As I grew, so did my passion for music and playing any instrument I could get my hands on. I practiced every day as long as I could during the rain, shine, night or day. When I was young music was a true passion for me.

My next passions came in high school as an athlete, playing both softball and basketball. I would never be the star. I devoted my life to running, weight lifting and health, to achieve and strengthen the incredible passion of winning. I loved the pride that came with a clutch hit or free throw. I could do this until my drenched, tired body said, "No more."

In college, my passion was softball, for it gave me a sense of direction and purpose. I had never thought I was smart enough to be a college student but here I was and I was succeeding.

It was not until I reached my postgraduate studies that I realized my greatest passion was my success at work as a contract specialist. It was so high that the potential loss of that would devastate my personality and zest for life. I used to get such a natural high when I was negotiating a contract, especially the ones where I knew I could win. I loved not knowing what the settlement would bring, what unexpected conditions or complications might arise. This was great! I would practice the negotiation in my dreams. It was a way to rehearse it before it took place. It is what I loved most. My career became increasingly important for me. It was not everything, but it was a very big part of my life. My success would reflect upon my children and their ability to succeed in life. I could give to them those things that they needed to be successful in everything they wanted to do. My success and my ability to give my children the opportunity to succeed were my life's goals.

When my children were born, my desire to make my mark increased twofold. I wanted my children to be proud of their mother's career. I needed to give them more than just clothes and piano lessons I wanted to give them pride. I wanted to be their example of hard work and determination.

I wanted to give them pride in their life and pride in their history.

I would soon learn that the stroke would destroy my passion for life, my passion for success and learning. I did not care anymore. My children would now have to fend for themselves. As bad as it sounds, at that point in my life I did not care.

Now the sermon on passion stuck with me. I really don't know why. Was it because he spoke about changing your passions? As I listened I realized that the stroke had not only changed me, my abilities, and the way I "see" but it had also changed my passions. I already had an incredible passion for people, but this passion would explode after the stroke. I have a deep need to be around and help others. Mainly, I love to learn and share with other stroke survivors.

I have found that my passion for my children has also changed. It's a passion for their emotional and physical heath. It's the passion for not giving them "things" but for teaching them about life. To teach them to love and have compassion for all people. I want to instill in them that merely making money and giving them "things" is not what makes us a parent. The best parents teach without the unnecessary commercial "stuff" of life. So my passion now lies in my spirit, in my ability to learn and help people, all people. So when I learn, it may be that the stroke is the hardest lesson in life. I have learned that with all things considered, even the bad, when the learning changes your passions it can change them to a better more enhanced fulfilled passion of life. My passion is quest for understanding the spirit of the human heart.

Coffee and Cream

As the dark stream of vanilla cream makes it's way to the bottom of the cup I see a reflection of me changing with each new creamy swell. I look back to see the pure cream that once dumped its calming smooth texture into my soul. Only now that the cream slowly fades into the dark rich grounds its sweetness is eroded. I try to add a taste full of sugar to calm its bite but the power the Java has is to strong. It is then that I realize that at some point in time, we are all like coffee and cream, trying to preserve our sweetness.

Grass

As I stand here and look back on my life, where I was and where I am going, I try to comprehend what my purpose really is. As I peer down to the ground, I notice that each blade of grass reaches to the sun in a different manner, each with it's own direction and understanding of what its real purpose is. Some say its purpose is to soften the blow of a toddler's foot as she runs barefoot across the lawn. Some say that it's to protect and nourish the earth. For some, it's just to protect its roots; for others it's to comfort the children as they roll along the way. Then there is one, a single blade that fights to find its purpose. The longer that blade fights, the more it seems to lose its strength, and until one day it cannot provide any insulation or protection to its roots. It can no longer protect and reach to the sun for warmth. At that point when all else has failed, it gives up and dies. So if we are like blades of grass and we each try to find our purpose, the one that fulfills our heart and soul, at that point, when purpose has gone or is no longer recognizable we slowly wither away. For just like grass, most plants grow productive and fruitful, providing the wheat that feeds us. But there are always some that seem to have life ahead that for some reason just start to wither away. As we look into our own eyes, is it not purpose that we all must find? For if we have no purpose, then we have no life.

When you have a stroke you lose your purpose. You didn't give it up its stripped away from you. After stroke each thing that you have learned and experience in your life before the stroke is now questioned. You feel as though you can not claim those things you had done because they were done as a "former self." Stroke makes you redefine and look for a new purpose. The purpose I was once comfortable with is now different. It has not changed but I have. When we change so does our purpose how ever slight that may or may not be. I can't count on those people, places and memories that I once had. I must first build a new self. Once I am somewhat comfortable with my new self I must then deal with my deficits and my limitations that accompany them. When I have tackled those three things my sense of self which brings confidence will give me a sense of worth. With a sense of worth I can find a new purpose. That purpose may be totally different than what it was before the stroke but it may also just be a better rendition of what it use to be. I believe that if we allow ourselves to learn that we can then smile and say we are lucky. We have the ability to correct what we have done wrong in the past for we are making a new person with a new life. We must find the purpose of who we are, why we are, and then be the best we can be with that purpose in mind. Stroke does not give you your purpose but it will let us find it for ourselves. There is nothing that defines our purpose it is up to us to define it, refine it, and share it with others. My purpose has evolved since I had my stroke. I have purpose in my job to show that I can conquer and still contribute. I have purpose to help people understand that stroke is not the end of us. We are even more worthy of life as we have survived. My main purpose is to make sure that my husband and children know and live in the love that I have for them. My purpose is still evolving and it will change with time as I change but one thing is for sure, I have more purposes now than I did before my stroke. I am very grateful for that.

Donna Brady

Panic

Panic

I panic at pain, I panic at loss, I panic at strength, and I panic in crowds. What is panic? Panic is the inability to fulfill your destiny, to reach to the stars and touch one. Panic makes me lost in a familiar place and lonely when others are around. Panic strikes when you least expect it with a vengeance of unknown proportions. To look at the familiar like you have never see it before. Panic makes you fight against the threat of not remembering. Panic is how you feel as you try to fight your way back to where you were when the end is nowhere in sight.

I had not experienced panic until after the stroke. I would often get nervous before a big game or a big briefing but I would never panic. Panic was for the weak at heart and weak in soul. I now was panicking at everything I tried to do. I was afraid to tell others until it was apparent that these attacks were not going to go away. It would take several uncontrollable occasions before I would realize that panic was an uncontrollable intense frustrating feeling of helplessness that can only be understood by those who have panicked. These occasions of panic mold the doubt that stroke has already left behind. The attacks seemed, for awhile, to just confirm the fact that I have no control over what had happened to my brain and my life. Since I now have the attacks under control, with medication and therapy, I have often wished that we all could understand more deeply how others with panic disorders feel without having to experience it. I now understand first hand the shame and depression that the attacks create.

Driving Again
(The First Attack I Remember)

Today is the day I decided that I would try to drive. I needed to regain my independence again. I longed for it in everything I did. I was very worried that I couldn't do it and that I would be like a lot of the other stroke survivors, dependent on others to get around. That thought alone was enough to depress me. I wasn't ready for face that too. I know my vision is getting better and I can see well enough to drive. I have to practice driving because in two short weeks I have to retake my driver's test. To read the words and comprehend them then select the right answers. Not only did I have to pass the vision test but I also had to be able to drive there. This is and of itself frightened me. I get so confused and scared these days. I lack the confidence to do and take actions on my own without direction. If I am to go back to work I must be able to drive. I want to take myself to therapy. I want to drive on my own. I hate being a burden to my husband who must help get me and our three children ready each Monday, Wednesday, and Friday so that I can go to therapy. They have to sit in the lobby for an hour while I try to relearn all those things I learned as a child. I really hate what this has done to us. It has taken away all that I have worked for and achieved.

I was really afraid that I couldn't do the written test. I talked to Christine about it. She helped me find a place that could re-teach me to drive. After hours of thinking about the next humiliation that would bring me to admit that there is yet another thing I can not do, I decided to first try it myself. So with the book in hand and hours of my sister reading it to me because I read way to slow to get this done in time I set off to retake the test on my own. My sister Karen tested me and supported me through out this nauseating ordeal. I left bright and early shaking like a leaf I kissed Mike goodbye. I was so nervous that I couldn't eat.

This was a test of my inner strength, my ability to once again face my fears of post-stroke failure. Well it only took one hour to read, comprehend, and answer the 15-question test, but I did it! It was all I could do not to explode with joy and embarrass myself in front of all those people. You would think I was a 16-year-old kid again. Ok now the vision test I hope that the right words come out when I have to read the signs. I was worried I would mess this up and have to tell them about me. It wasn't seeing the signs that scared me it was the words that might force their way through my lips. What and how would I explain that I know it's a stop sign when the word said, "banana." It's the aphasia that said, "A candy bar." I rehearsed and rehearsed the signs everyday, saying the words out load over and over. I would draw the letters of the signs on paper over and over again. During the test I would draw the signs in my hand before I would answer to help make sure I would say the right word. I'm sure that the lady at the counter thought I was really weird. Christine taught me rehearse it, see it, feel it, and say it and I would be better prepared to remember it. Remember you use your sight, ears, and voice to communicate. Use all of these to communicate if you need too. Thank goodness I remembered what she had taught me. I passed the test! I can't believe it! I was so happy that when I walked to my car I collapsed and cried for what seemed to be an eternity. I can't believe I did it! Why are these things so hard for me to do? Why? I still don't really understand all of this.

I told Christine I passed the test. I told her how long it took but how much time didn't seem to matter. She said, "I knew you would do it." She had more confidence in me than I did. I looked at her smile for approval each time I did a task. I needed confirmation that I was doing things right. I do not trust the answers my brain gives me. This lack of trust in my abilities haunts me day in and day out. I often wonder what abilities I will have from day to day. The constant state of questioning my own abilities and choices would cause the panic to reach a new height when I returned to work. I had never had a panic attack before this but then I had never had a stroke either. It may now take me years to learn but I do learn. It's better to learn slowly than not at all. It wouldn't be for many months that I would realize that the me I was trying to achieve wasn't really there anymore. I was trying to be an unachievable person who had become a memory with the stroke.

Lost in the crowd
(The Second Attack I remember)

Today was the day I would attempt to go Christmas shopping with my oldest child April. We were both very excited as it had been months since we had been anywhere alone together. We had been missing out on a big part of each other's life. Since the stroke I have been out of touch. I had no real idea of what she thought and how she felt. We talked sometimes but she was afraid and I wasn't capable of really listening.

Our day started off by taking the Jimmy to the mall. I would learn later that I should have started off in a less intense area for our first post-stroke adventure together. The drive was uneventful. We parked and walked hand in hand swinging our way past the doors to Hudson's. We like Hudson's it is a very nice entrance to a very big place.

Ok April where do we start? What do you want to do? What do you want to get for Amber and Daddy? "What about Alexa," she said. I had forgotten for a moment that I had three children. Well since she is a baby we'll go to Toys-R-Us for her ok? "Sure mom, that sounds good," she said with a smile. Let's get Amber's presents from Toys-R-Us too. It was set we were on our adventure. We would try to do lunch and shopping for dad. As we walked out of Hudson's into the mass of busy shoppers bumping into each other I was filled with a sense of anticipation. It was so beautiful with all the Christmas tree's, wrapped gifts under the tree's, and children lined up to see Santa. We hurried to find our place in the driving hoards of people. Our first stop was Sears. What more does a man need? Tool belt and leather jacket. Ok we're off! The tool belt was first. April said, "I really want to get him the one like Uncle Paul's." That way daddy can hang his hammer from his belt, and then he doesn't have to keep climbing up and down the ladder each time he needs it. With that we were off for a handy man's tool belt. There are hundreds she said. Mommy which one do you like? Good question I really didn't know. All the crowds of people and noise were already overwhelming me. I couldn't handle the whining kids; it made me angry, and hurt my head. I like them all I said to her, it's your gift you pick the one you like best I am sure he'll love it. Ok but I can't decide between this one and that one, as she held two belts exactly the same just of a different hue in color. April it's up to you honey. Mom I want you to help me. An intense sense of needing to escape came over me. My 8-year-old daughter was demanding an answer and I didn't have one. I was so panicked that I couldn't think well enough to really know what she was asking. It was a simple decision she wanted me to help her make but I couldn't. She wanted some type of decision from me and I couldn't offer it. Right at that moment a lady bumped into me. She scowled at me and it made me feel incredibly small it was like she could see that I wasn't normal anymore. Mom which one? Oh, um that one. I just put my hand out and pointed into the general direction. "The light one I like it too," she said as she smiled. We were past that thank goodness. I was ready to leave. April didn't even know how overwhelmed I was. She was just happy to be with me.

    Mom I really want a drink. Ok good idea I am thirsty too. We walked out of Sears and found a place to get a pop.

When I Learn . . .Surviving Stroke with Pride

I need to go to the bathroom mom. Why didn't you go before we left? Mom I didn't have to go then. April I don't know where the bathroom is from here. We passed one at Hudson's, she said. I was panicked at this point. I didn't know if I could stay in this crowd much longer. We would have to walk all the way to Hudson's for her to use the restroom then all the way back to Sears. As we made our way back to Hudson's I remember from my previous years of mall shopping that all department stores have restrooms. I should have known, how stupid of me! I hate this! I really hate my brain now. Learn it again Donna that's all you can do. Hopefully I learn it faster than I learned to read. As we ventured through the mass back to Sears I asked April if she would mind if we finished another day. No! Mom you promised! That I had and I couldn't break it. We had both looked forward to it for some time. We proceeded even with my resentment of having to feel this way. Why am I feeling this? My chest is hurting and my head is pounding. Am I going to have another stroke right here? Please don't let me get sick here. I don't want April to go through that again.

As we walked I asked her how school was going. She said all right. I asked her if anything was bothering here as I had gotten a call from her teacher asking me if things were ok at home. Mom, my teacher doesn't like me. I don't know why. The teacher had remarked that April is a wonderful child who doesn't listen well. April when your teacher asks you a question are you concentrating on the answer? Yes mommy as hard as I can. I just forget. Why do you think you forget? I don't know. How are your friends? I don't have any friends. What do you mean, I thought you were playing with Lilly and Mary. They don't like me anymore. They told me I couldn't play with them because of the first graders. What do you mean? I play with the first graders who don't have friends, the new kids. What do you think about them not wanting you to play with the first graders? I think they are wrong. I think we should play with everyone.

I think they are mean. You're right honey we shouldn't ever not play with someone because they are younger or different but you should also play with people your own age. Mom? Yes hon. You know there is a boy at school he says he can't play with me because you are handicapped. He says your stupid. Are you stupid? What do you think April? Isn't stupid a bad word? That's what you told me mom right? Yes April. Do you think I am stupid? No I think your smart, you're really smart because you can read and write again. It hit me really hard like a ton of bricks. It was at that moment walking through the mall that I realized that my stroke did more than just take from me but it took a part of them too. My family has suffered as I have. I just looked at her and hugged her tight. I said, "I love you April." "I love you too mommy," she said. I told him you're a 100% now but he didn't believe me! You're not stupid at all! That's good hon. April? Yes mom. I am very proud of you. You make sure you tell Mommy if anyone ever says anything to hurt you ok? Ok. You promise? "Yes," she said with a smile.

Well here we were back at Sears. A single leather coat is why we were enduring this pain. Pain I am so sick of it. I am really tired. My legs and feet are starting to hurt and I can feel a headache coming on. Damn it Donna, you have to do this your promised. Donna stop thinking of yourself, think of April. Think of how long she has waited for this day. The walk took a lot out of me but it was intensified by what was going on with my daughter. I felt guilty that she ever had to go through this. Well we finally reached Sears and got to the coat rack and after a few moments selected what we thought to be the coolest coat possible for Mike. Mm I love the smell of leather. The lady comes to help us since the coat is attached to the rack by a long locked cable. Let me get the keys for you. Now the last thing I needed was for them to lose those keys. It will be a moment we have to get the manager to bring her set of keys. How long

When I Learn . . .Surviving Stroke with Pride

will that take? Only a moment mam I am sorry for the inconvenience. I was getting to my end, that point where I was going to lose control. I couldn't have a panic attack here in front of April. She could already sense that I was on the edge because I was getting very hyper with her. I wanted to get out of there. I started pacing a little trying to get rid of this excess energy that was building up inside of me but it was just coming to fast. I saw the lady and she said another minute. I told her I could come back she said now she'll be here. Well minutes and hours seemed to pass and I was ready to get out of there. I need to get out of the noise, the lights, the smell and the closing of the walls around me. April and I chit chatted about nothing really. I tried to focus on her, Christmas and our plans for a great holiday. I went to the counter again to find the lady that was helping me. They told me she left for her lunch break. I was hot I was boiling inside with anger. Is this customer service? I have been standing here for almost an hour waiting for those keys and I am really getting tired of this. Hundreds of people have been helped. The lady, a bit startle at my reaction, started to look at me and pulled the keys out of the drawer. I don't know why she didn't see them. I will help you immediately mam, I am sorry. She didn't tell me you were here waiting on the keys. The manager came up at that moment. She asked who paged her. I told her what happened. I am sorry she's new here. I didn't want to buy the coat then but I had been there so long that I couldn't leave without it. I paid for the coat and we left. I was mad, my head hurt and I hated life at that moment. Why do we do this to ourselves year after year! April wanted to stop at a few more stored. I told her, I am sorry honey but mommy isn't feeling well is it ok if we leave? Ok Mommy. As we got outside of Hudson's into the fresh cold air I started feeling better and less confined. I really treasure the quiet now. I'm not fit for the hustle and bustle of what my former life brought. I still don't want to admit that I have changed so dramatically. This too will pass I told myself. I told myself to remember that the first time I do something it will be scary but then it will get easier. You're just retraining your brain. That's all it is, refreshing your new self.

The Airport

It is my first trip for work. Oh my God I think I am going to pass out. I am so frightened of what is going to happen at the airport that I can't sleep that night. Thank you lord for letting Carol be so nice. She gave me a ride to the airport so I didn't have to worry about driving on that bad road where no one seems to care about your life more or less theirs. I would have to give myself several extra hours to get ready for the trip because I lost my self in the packing activities and more often than not didn't realize what it was I had started out to do. Once in the car heading for the airport I found myself staring at the clock wondering when we were going to get there. I always give myself an extra hour depending on where I am going. Just in case I forget. I was worried about getting there because it seems to be taking so long although in reality it was only a half an hour. My heart was racing almost the entire way. I hoped I give Mike my plan numbers just in case. I feared falling from the sky. I would much rather end my own life than fall to my death. I think it would be easier for the kids if I died in an accident than by my own hands. Problem with that is others might try to save me in an accident. I can not go through this again. I really hate what the stroke did to me.

Carol was telling me about her dog chasing the rabbits in her back yard. The rabbit and dog are fine. I wish I could run away from this intense sensation I am feeling about this trip. I am totally petrified of this week. I am going to a place I know I know but don't really feel like I remember. I have been envisioning the terminals that we will walk through, put on my fanny pack so I don't forget my purse, and tickets. We are finally here; the lady is really perturbed about where we parked how simple her life is to be angry over our choice of parking spots. She made us move the car. How stupid I thought, then she said we'd mess up their system if we walk across the street. I then understood because I had a system for parking my Jimmy at work so that I could always find it. Get there really early park at the end next to the red gravel.

We're at the airport and we checked our luggage in. I let Carol go first so I could copy her. I did not want anyone to know I felt lost and completely out of control. My blood pressure I though would give me away because I felt it was so high that my eyes had to be bulging from their sockets. Can't they see the terror I feel right at this moment? We talked endlessly about this and that I don't recall the exact conversation. I remember writing my seat number on my hand. Row 10 seat A by the window so I wouldn't forget. I just prayed that I could read the number once I got on the plane. I held my tickets into my hands as we walked down the breezeway. I took a deep breath and said a prayer as I sat down and buckled my seat belt. I looked forward concentrating on my tickets and hoping that the guy sitting next to me couldn't hear my rapid breathing. God get me through this. "Don't let me die here," I kept saying over and over and over. It was that second when the jet engine roared that all I had been through this year started racing through my mind. It was a culmination of happiness, sadness, fear, turmoil, pain and anger. Oh God I wish I were sitting in her office she'd know what to do. Too late your here just don't let them know don't let them see what your feel. Swallow the confusion and panic, smile and most of all concentrate on your eyes. Remember your eyes give away to all your moods and your personality. Whew were up. No thanks I am not thirsty or hungry. If she only knew I would throw up if I even touched my lips to anything. I tried to do homework Christine gave me but couldn't. I am looking at it and realize I don't know what I am supposed to do. I fake it by scribbling what appears to be some notes and put it away. Look like you're tired and try to sleep. I closed my eyes and concentrated and kept telling myself, "Think like you are in your car sitting on the ground. Hell Donna, I-696 is this bumpy. I don't panic when I'm a passenger on the ground so why am I panicking now? The captain comes on we are landing in a few moments thank you for flying with us today. If your gate information is not in the list we have two people as you get off the plane to get you on your way to your next scheduled flight for those of you who are continuing on. I heard no more I just kept thinking, "Thank goodness we are half way there." I remember them saying Ft. Walton beach on Concourse B. We were landing in A. My heart started racing again. I hope I don't lose Carol. We landed which gave me a big sense of relief that I was on the ground again. I got off and waited for Carol. I was thankful that I remember that she was in the back of the plane. There she is. "A smooth flight huh?," I muttered. She said, "yes." One down one to go I said with a smile. Ok we need to go to B the man pointed us in the right direction. Off we go. Oh my God look at all these people. Can they tell I am not normal? I stayed with Carol until I saw the Body Works shop. I was almost out of lotion and peered into the window. I forgot that I was walking with Carol. I look up and she was no where to be seen. Oh shit what do I do now? Panic of indescribable proportions engulfed my brain, my stomach, my chest, my legs and my hands. I tried to remember where I was going, what we came in on, A gate to B, no wait was it in on B leaving on A? Oh Donna calm yourself down you have done this before. She'll meet you there. You can do this; you have done it a thousand times before. Yes I have but it was before the stroke. I kept trying to psyche myself into calmness. You can do this. Oh my what if I miss my flight? I didn't know what any of the answers were to my brains spinning questions. What do I do? Call Mike? Call Connie? I can't call anyone because then they will know how bad all of this really is for me. Get a grip. Stare at the window and put yourself together. There are monitors that tell you where to go, but I can't read them they are to high and small. Oh know what am I going to do? Why is this happening to me?

Call Christine, she'll know what to do. I don't have her phone number and I can't call her either. Dam you can't run to her every time you have a stroke problem. Therapy is over Donna get it through your thick head you have to help yourself. A tap on my shoulder with a "Donna I lost you" brought me back to reality. It was Carol, I smiled and said "Oh I'm sorry, I am out of lotion and I thought they might have it. Sorry. She had to have noticed the energy drainage from my face because I could feel stinging of swat against my cheeks.

We have to go she said. Boy there are a lot of people aren't' there? Yes, imagine what it was like during the Olympics. To busy for me I said. We got to our next flight. The plane was small but at least it is a jet. I was so thankful that Carol had the rental car. I took a deep breath while we were going to the hotel. I asked her, "Do you know what I hate?" "I get turned around easily." I do too, she said. I told her that I was glad she was driving. The less pressure on me the better I thought. She said it's ok it's your first time away since your stroke. Don't worry your fine. She is a kind thoughtful person. I'm lucky she works with me.

It often takes me awhile to learn. This trip taught me that others would help even if I didn't try to hide my deficits. People do care but we have to let them. It is those people that have compassion that will not leave you stranded. I know that there is always going to be people that don't care but the ones that do far out-weigh the ones that don't. Those people that don't care just need to learn themselves.

I have been fighting for some time now to get rid of the panic that takes control of my emotions and my body. I would not learn until months later that sometimes there is nothing emotionally you can do to control it. It is OK to ask for help with all these things. Panic is an outcome of a horrible experience and violation of your brain called "stroke". I have learned now that we must all go though the stages to learn and regain our life. Nothing worth having is ever easy.

Hiding

I was sitting here at my computer today wondering if there is some point in time that my thoughts would just stop. That my days would not be filled with stroke questions of why me and how. What causes it and why did it happen to me? I went to a wedding with my husband last night. It was a lot of fun we socialized with people we don't get to see that often.

When we entered the room that was packed with about two hundred people I took Mike by the hand and told him don't leave me behind. It is all so overwhelming for me at first. The music and bustle of all the relatives greeting each other with hugs and kisses was overpowering me. I often wonder if they can see my nervousness as we start to greet each other. We found Mike's mom and I planted myself next to her. I could just sit there. People were talking to me but I couldn't hear them. It was really loud but it was hard for me to concentrate on their words. I often have no control over which voice or sound gets my attention.

I am getting to be a pro at hiding my deficits. I am slowly learning that is not a good thing. I have cost myself some valuable learning and time because of pride and honor. It is quite strange that out of all these people there is one that always seems to see when I am hiding. Trying to act normal when I feel so abnormal. Maybe it is the look in my eyes or the expression on my face, I do not know, but I know that whatever it is she senses it and always seems to save me.

I was sitting there trying to act interested in the conversation but I was having a hard time keeping up with the words, their voices, and their gestures. In small social situations or when the noise level is low I have no problems. I get my reminders when I am out of control of the situation. I think that is why I can still speak in front of others as long as I receive no blind-sided question. The disk jockey decided it was time to get the pace up and lights on high. The strobe lights were making me dizzy, the music was hurting my head, and my throat was hurting from trying to hear myself talk. It is quite funny how in order to remember my conversation and where I am that I need to hear myself talk. That revelation came to me recently at work when the noise level was so high that I was getting very annoyed and agitated. It was bad enough that it forced me to leave for a while so that my co-workers would not see me over react from the stress. I was at the point already and we had only gotten there maybe thirty minutes ago. Then she came over.

Donna how are you? I am fine how are you doing? "Good," she said. So how are things really going? She always seems to know when I am having a hard time getting words and keeping my concentration. She asked me how my speech to the stroke club went, and I told her better than I expected. I told her I really enjoyed it. It was nice meeting others who are going and have been going through this. I told her about the book I had just read and she was interested. She's a nurse, I am not sure how many people like me she knows but she seems eager to understand. She is very patient with me and always makes me feel good. She even laughs at my corny jokes.

I entitled this portion of the chapter hiding because I find that I try to hide behind what others knew about me before I had my stroke. I don't want to be judged on who I am after the stroke because at this point I had not accepted the person the stroke left me with. It is amazing that I find that I now appreciate the new me much more than the old one even thought I still don't really accept her as my own. To hide behind a previous life is very difficult. When you slip people see how the stroke affected you. Since you have been hiding their reaction are often worse because you weren't up front with them early on. I think it makes them feel as though you don't trust them when in facts it's that I don't trust who I am.

Now that I have learned to talk about the stroke and my deficits I find most people are willing to accept and be patient with me. Those people who are not accepting and not patient are not worth my energy and chose not to understand. I find now that because of the stroke people like seeing me around it reminds them about how important life is and how easily it is taken. Someone said to me once, "Each time I look at you I can see how good God can be when all is felt to be lost". "You remind me of how strong our sprits are when we want them to be". "You remind me how unimportant certain things really are". I told her, "Family, faith and life are important, money and "stuff" isn't". I can live without the stuff but I can't live without family, friends and faith. So when I learn often others do too, if I let them.

Help Me

Admitting is hard

I made the call today. After months of contemplation I finally decided that I needed help. The nightmares, the panic attacks and the feeling of suicide keeps me from enjoying life. I had opportunities by the number to either make the call or end my life but I just couldn't do it, I could not do either one. I told myself that both would be selfish. My kids deserve a stable and alive mother. I thought that neither a psychologist nor suicide offered me what I needed. I just wanted me back. I already knew I was crazy. People my age don't want to kill themselves. I didn't need someone to reconfirm what I already knew. The stroke had already taken so much away from me that admitting yet another failure was more than I could bear. I needed help learning to accept my limitations, my disabilities and my new me. I needed to understand that I had lost the old Donna but that the one who took her place was also good.

It was a bad day I had been up all night with the nightmares. Each time I would drift off to sleep I would be awaken by my heart racing, my sweat drenched nightgown and in a state of panic. I would be breathing so rapidly I couldn't believe that Mike didn't hear it. I would sit up afraid to fall asleep again because of the terrors I would endure. To relive and relive over and over the process of dying.

Most of the dreams were of loss and confusion. Being lost and not finding my way. Being caught by a bandit in the night that keeps ripping at my abilities. Other dreams centered on my deficits and not being able to recover from them. The fear I would feel of having another stroke only this time I didn't recover so well. Being afraid of losing my family because I couldn't be a contributing provider to our household as I have always been. The reality that I could lose my job and knowing that no one else would hire me. Finally thinking that if I was to end my life they would be better off. They would have enough money to go to school, get a great house and be happy.

The nightmares would start as a simple dream. Like going to work. I would be in a meeting giving a presentation lose the words. Everyone would start looking at me then they start laughing, they shake their head, they yell get out, your are not fit, you are not fit for living! In one of the nightmares I was paralyzed from the neck down having a stroke during the night. I yelled as hard as I could but my voice was no where to be found. Mike he is right next to me. How can I get his attention? I can't move, my body is frozen and I am a prisoner in my own head. I will die! My breath is hard and labored. I will suffocate here next to him without him knowing. The kids, what happens if they find me? My heart is pounding, my breathing is rapid and my entire body is fighting to move! I am panicking I feel the heat in my chest, the pressure in my heart, I can hear it, it is beating so fast that I can't even breath well enough to slow it down. God! It's really happening! I can't believe that now it will happen again after all this, after all of this rehabilitation and therapy and trying to get better. To do and be who I was. Why are you letting this happen to me now? Why now? Please answer me! No! I scream out loud and I sit up like a rocket shot high into the heaven. I can barely even focus on where I am. What is happening? My arms are shaking, my legs are weak and I can't breath. Oh my God it was a dream! Mike, he's still at work, it's only 11:30PM I have only been sleeping for an hour. I don't want to fall asleep. I hate sleeping. It's a double edge sward. If I don't sleep I can't talk well, get words or function. If I do sleep, I wake up three to four times a night from nightmares. This one was so bad that it woke up April so I decided it was time. Swallow your pride and make the call. I can not do this by myself anymore. I had talked to Christine about it a few times. She thought it would be a good idea and gave me the number to call. She had no idea of what was really happening. Had I been strong enough to tell her, I would have saved myself a lot of pain, I know that now. The one thing I didn't lose was my self-conscious behavior and perceptions of what therapy especially psychological therapy means. Misconception or not, I thought it would mean that I was an unstable person who could not handle my own problems and my own life. Everyone has problems so why couldn't I now handle my own? That means I am crazy. If I need a psychologist that is admitting that I can't handle it myself. I am not strong, stable, or sane. I have always been the stable force, the one others could lean on, I was not us to nor had I ever had to lean on others before.

The call was hard. I was scared, nervous and worried. It was all I could do to even talk that day. I made the call and after being transferred from one place to another I had three numbers. The first one was not a provider of my insurance. So why was it that my insurance is the one that gave me that number? I almost decided not to try. I tried to talk myself into thinking I can deal with this myself. I sat the phone down then thought long and hard about the dreams and not being able to get the stroke out of my mind. Ok, I will call this number but that's it. I would not call another number if this one doesn't work. Then at least I can say I tried. I dialed the phone and a message service came on line. Doctor's answering service may I help you? Um yes I guess. Um my insurance gave me her number. She is not available at this moment can I have her call you? I guess so. I need your name and phone number please. I gave it to her. To my surprise I received a call from the doctor herself in what seemed to be minutes. My time that day was at a stand still. That day took forever. She asked me why I had called. I thought to myself "Ok Donna, truth time now." I am 35 years old, I had a stroke 15 months ago and I keep having nightmares and panic attacks. Well Ms. Brady I would really like to take you as a patient but I am full right now. My heart started sinking. Denial set in. Did the insurance give you any other names? Yes but they are really far away. I don't like driving where I am not familiar. I have a small vision problem from the stroke. I don't read well so I like staying in my own area if I can. Well I'll tell you what, you can either call the other therapist who may be able to get you in faster or I can see you but you have to understand that it would be as my appointment schedule will allow. I am filled so I can't promise regular appointments. What would you like to do? Um. I don't know. Take your appointments I guess. I won't call anyone else. I told her I had three kids then asked her if she had any children. She has three kids herself. I know I like her already. I knew I wouldn't call another because this was one of the hardest phone calls I have ever had to make. I even went as far as promising Christine I would call so that I had to try. I wouldn't break a promise to Christine so I knew when I hit the send button I had to make at least one call. I don't lie and not to lie meant I had to call. I would not break a promise to her I knew that. So when I hit send I made a promise that I had to fulfill. Ok, can you come in next week Thursday at 11AM? Yes I can. Try to be 15 minutes early to fill out paper work. I was 25 minutes early because I was afraid of how long it would take me to fill out the forms.

Now I am becoming an old pro at this therapy stuff. I haven't had a nightmare in months. I am no longer afraid to fall asleep. I do not get the panic attacks as often either. She has helped give me perspective. I know that what I feel and what I am experiencing is normal for what I have been through. I am really normal! I am also learning to like the new me a little at a time. That it's ok to feel sad about losing who you were but you have to find who you are now and like that person to survive. Time is our friend and we must embrace it with all our energies. For time helps us see the light when the tunnel looks so dark. I am glad that I made that phone call. I have only one regret now and that is that I didn't tell Christine all of what was happening to me. I probably have more deficits that she could have helped me with but I let my own selfish pride get in the way. I should have made the phone call earlier. I wish that a stroke came with a help file like MS Word it would save a lot of energy. It would be nice to have a brain center to access when your lost and don't know where to go but I would want it to have a great search capability. I also think that it is sad that we have allowed ourselves to be misled about what is "normal" and "stable." Needing to talk to someone to gain understanding and perspective is a good thing not a bad thing.

Mental Medication

Well today was the day that I would finally admit to myself that I can't do it alone. That I am no longer strong enough to work my way back to me. Med.'s are what they are referred to by stroke survivors. Some are on blood thinners that could make you bleed but prevent stroke. Some are on heart pills to keep their life pumping to a rhythm. While others are on antidepressants, panic attack and sleeping pills to sustain a normal mental life.

I told myself I would not become a victim of the brain killers. That to limit my ability to think and react through medication was limiting me as a person. That giving in to drugs was not an answer. That all things good and bad could be learned and handled with training. I have been trying to train my brain to act like it us to, to react normally. To think before it reacts. I have now found that after eighteen months of training I am tired. Tired of fighting to keep and get back what I lost. Tired of hurting inside everyday. Sick of feeling sick and not being normal.

My anger and mood swings scare me. I don't know why it happens but it doesn't take much to set me off ranting and raving. I haven't hit my kids but I yell at them. They don't deserve to be yelled at each day because I can't deal with my own problems. It's not their fault that all this has happened and there is nothing they can do about it. My bursts of anger now scare me to the point that for my children as well as myself I will succumb to the brain medication. I will reach to them for help in gaining self-control and understanding of who I am now. This decision makes me feel weak and less of a person inside. It makes me feel like I will some how become just another junky who needs drugs to survive.

I know that this is not the same. My intellectual self tells me it will help me keep control. It will chemically allow me to obtain a little more of my former self. I need balance in my life and this was the way to get to it. I was banking on that it would somehow help me return back to me.

Some med.'s are good I know that. The ones that keep my heart beating help my body sustain my life. Why is it that when it comes to medication for our soul or sanity in life that we resist so hard? We find it easy to swallow antibiotics when we are physically ill but when our pain comes from our emotions we find swallowing difficult.

Is it not our physical brain that was harmed during the stroke? If so then the mental pain is only a reflection of our brains physical sense to health. We physically see and feel our arms, legs and hands. It is our emotional pain that the brain feels. For if emotional pain was not physically born then we would have control of our emotional and mental wellbeing with no regard for the physical being. I feel the changes in me. My emotional side hurts, it aches for relief. My dreams ache for relaxation and my mood for comfort. Maybe these med.'s will help my brain. Help it find peace again. Find the peace that I once had before the stroke took so much from me.

Always thinking mentally

1. Thank you for taking me as a patient. I know that you have a waiting list. I do appreciate it.
2. I have been thinking a lot lately, as my brain never stops. It is always dreaming and thinking. Some thoughts are good but some are bad.
3. I still don't know why the stroke has changed me so dramatically. Why my thoughts and perceptions of

life and it's purpose were lost. It seems that it's started to fade. It's like I am slowly but surely dying inside. That the person I had worked so hard to create was taken away from me before she was allowed to enjoy the benefits of that labor.

4. You said that you could read between the lines of my booklet I wrote. What did you see?

5. I think about the stroke, about the new disk that has blown in my neck, about the mass they found in my stomach that just seems to disappear after 6 months, about the monthly problems, and my emotional state.

6. One thing I do know for sure that the stroke changed me. The only part of me that did not change is my love and caring for people. Yet although I have that now I care so much and love so much that it hurt all the time. I worry about things I have no control over to the point that I get physically sick. I do things not just once but 3 or 4 times over because I don't trust myself. I worry about what I say and if I made anyone angry. I can't handle people being angry with me...therefore I give in despite what I think.

7. I am angry now and I have never been an angry person. I use to pride myself on being able to forgive and forget. I yell a lot. I put myself in time out but I don't have control of my emotions and I don't know why. They tell me and all the stroke group survivors say that is a part of the brain injury loss of emotional control. I say that I have to have control so that I can teach my kids well for the only chance they have is me. If I can't give them that chance then my existence is more worth less than I thought.

8. I am depressed all the time and that just keeps grinding on me. I am happy one minute just to feel

the pit of my stomachache wanting to throw in the towel. I must be in some type of self-pity problem but I don't know how it started and I don't know how to stop it. Look at me I am functioning and working. Yes it is hard but so many can't even do that. Why in the heck do I feel this way! Why can't I stop it…I have to stop it….I feel like I am slowly dying inside that with each day I give up just a little more…eventually nothing will be left. Maybe that's good. If there is nothing to look forward to then all these bad things can't hurt me anymore.

9. You asked me if I was a spiritual person. Yes I am, was, not really sure now. I was a person who was going to make a different. Going to make this world a little better. My only thought in life was that at my grave to have just one person say that they were better off for having known me. That is what I strive for. I wanted to give my kids the best of life.

10. You said that maybe we should work on me liking me. I don't know how to do that anymore. How do you like someone you don't trust or wouldn't even want to know. I don't understand why or how the stroke could just take all I have worked for and throw it down the toilet. To be told, live with it. You look fine. You are blessed. You are lucky. It could be worse. You're doing great.

11. Now you ask why did I type this? Because my short-term memory is so bad that I wouldn't remember it and if I did it wouldn't come out right because the words are so hard to find now. So, what do you see? Not the person everyone else sees I bet. Can you see that person that others say is dynamic, strong, exciting and full of energy? The one that is always told "you're amazing." I have been searching for that person for months now…and I still haven't found her. Maybe you can help me do

that. Get another part of life back that I lost on Feb. 21, 1997.

When I learn it often comes with change. Change is often good even when it hurts. The person that others use to see is really still here but just in a new shell of life. I have learned that coming to terms with accepting the changes in personality and pride may often be confusing and very difficult but there is still that dynamic, strong, exciting and full of energy person, I just couldn't see it for I had not accepted the change in me. As I look back at this now I realize that a part of the old me still forms the self of the new me. My former is the guardian angel of the new self I have found for that angel has learned two life session by living two lives.

Anger

It was not until Christine asked me if I yell at the kids that the thought that I could get angry occurred to me. I was not angry about having a stroke at first that came much later. In the hospital when I got angry it was because I thought that I was fine. I needed to go home.

The anger started slowly deep down inside of me. Like a small seed that is hungry to grow so to the anger was hungry. I pushed it down each time telling myself that to be angry was not an option. It would start with a harmless comment here or there by an unsuspecting friend. At first it would come and go before I really noticed it. I would only know it was there because of the feeling it gave me deep down in my gut. I know one thing for sure and that is anger is like a seed that is growing. Its roots get stronger as it starts to take over the plants that surround it until one day it pushes itself above the ground not letting anything stop it. Anger is like that too. It grows each time you feed it by pushing it back down. With each push the anger intensifies and starts to slowly boil.

Donna Brady

I remember the first time I got really angry. It was a conversation with my husband. He told me that I hadn't done something that I swear I did. One problem with short-term memory is that I don't realize when I make a mistake because I don't remember it. My anger started with a simple "I know I did it" then escalated to "Don't tell me I didn't I know I did" and finally resulted in us being so made at each other that he would go to the bedroom to get out of the line of fire. The anger demon just kept growing inside of me.

I clenched my fists and gritted my teeth. I would not give in. Not until the anger was so intense and out of control that I wanted to die. I have never experienced anger like this before. It's almost a rage that takes control. It was at that point after Mike had left the room that the anger took possession of my soul. I hate what happened to me! I hate who I am now! I hate my life! I just hate it all! My clenched fist found its way to the kitchen cabinet. I hit it once and that was all it took. One single moment of losing control. I hit the cabinet so hard that I thought I broke my hand. That did not stop me. I had become accustomed to pain. To live with pain and to not know what a pain free life is. As I hit the cabinet for yet the fifth or sixth time I kept telling myself that I shouldn't be doing this. I shouldn't be doing this but I can't stop. I hope I hurt myself. I was to die! Eventually hitting my fist wasn't enough so I started pounding my head against he cabinet. If I couldn't remember I would beat it out of my brain or I would die. I wanted to die. The part of me that always had control had vanished. I did not stop hitting my swollen fists to the cabinet until Mike, startled at what he saw, stopped me. What are you trying to do hurt yourself? Yes, I don't care anymore! I just don't care it's not worth it! Not anymore!

He had never ever seen me angry like this before. He had never really heard me raise my voice. There in front of him stood someone he did not know. His wife was never angry not like this. I was always in control I know how to handle situations but that was now gone. Thank goodness the kids didn't see that. What would they think? I now feel like a bad mother because of my anger at life. How can I be good to them if I am not good to myself?

My inability to control my temper, my mood swings, my words and thoughts made me even more angry. It made me hate the fact that I had to go through this. I resented that it was me who had been damaged and I was not a bad person. Why do bad things happen to good people? Each day I am reminded of those things I can not do nor control anymore. Someone asked me how do you keep from being angry about it? I told her you don't. You get angry, you experience the hate and frustration of the situation you react, you over react and finally after what seems to be an eternity you consciously fight to get control. At first you don't really realize what is happening. It's in control before you have had a chance to stop it. It's not the mental part of the anger that you don't recognize its the physical take over of your heart racing, your blood pressure so high you think you'll burst, and the hyperness in each crevice of your body fighting to get out. That pure surge of adrenaline is what scares me.

It is quite amazing that until the stroke I had known people who got angry. People who lost control in seeming small situation that had no real impact on life itself. I couldn't understand how they could let themselves lose control. I know now the frustration and how weak you feel when you lose control despite what you're trying to tell yourself.

I have learned through many days of frustration that I can have some control, at least enough to get myself in my own internal or external time out if need to. To consciously remove myself from the situation that is making me angry.

Getting angry is healing as long as we do not hurt others in the process. Working through anger is refreshing but accepting and conquering your anger is exhilarating.

Conquering the anger over stroke and what it has taken from you and left behind is a process that takes time. I thought that once I was done with speech rehabilitation that I would be me again but it wasn't like that. I traded my emotional self healing for learning how to read, write, speak and remember. I push away Christine's attempts to get me to help my feelings of who I was. Mental therapy was not in my plan. What I have learned is that it is normal to be angry over the loss of abilities and your former self. It is normal to hurt for those things you once could do but now can't. I have also learned that the anger I feel inside is not the same anger that others feel. That I must always find out what it was that made me angry. Was it what they said? How they said it? Was it simply the fact that it reminded me of who I use to be but can't have? Anger is good as long as you use it to better who you are and why you are. I must take control over my anger and use it to learn. When I learn the better I am to you and to me. I have taken my anger to a new level. I have taken it to one that gives me the strength to say, "Yes, I had a stroke, I conquered my stroke and it changed me but I am a better person for it." I use that anger to research the possibilities of helping others and letting others know what frustration we live in. I want to make sure that others know its not just that we are angry people which we have the right to be but people motivated through anger to fight for who we are now and who we want to be.

Depression

Depression, what is depression? What does it mean to be depressed? Depression to me is to watch your life vanish in front of your eyes. I would say that depression is the art of taking your soul and converting it into darkness.

It was a bright warm day when she gave me the test results. I remember the sun was shining so bright I had to wear my sunglasses. It was cool enough that I had to wear

When I Learn . . .Surviving Stroke with Pride

my leather coat. I wore the one I purchased in San Francisco after the biggest most successful negation I had ever had. Maybe not the most successful in some terms but in the strength of my ability. I would learn this day that it would forever remain my best.

I walked in and sat down. I knew immediately she had the test results because I had been asking about them each session since the testing had been completed. I thought the tests would prove my point, that therapy was silly in my case. I was going back to work. She sat down more quietly than usual. A strange sense came over me. My stomach turned into knots as she stared at the paper and said, "I have the results." Do you want me to read them to you? Yes. Not realizing how that single answer would change my life, my concept of self and self worth, and my willingness to live forever. To this point I blamed my inability to read, my memory loss and inability to write words on my loss of eyes site. After all if I could see I could do all those things.

She asked me again if I wanted for her to read them. I said yes. She replied, "Are you sure?" I nodded yes again. I still had no idea of what she was trying to prepare me for. I did not even get the visual cues. Her quiet demeanor, her not opening the books we had been working on, and asking me twice if she should read them to me. All of these should had been all I needed to know that it wasn't what I expected. There were no pencils on the table I always use pensile in therapy. I should have recognized the behavior. It's the same anticipation that you get when you open the door and there stands a police officer. You hope it's just the neighbor kid busted your car window with a softball, not that a loved one was in an car accident.

She started reading. It took two sessions to finish. After the first page of words like Ms. Brady can't do, deficits, inability, not recognize, not perform, and decrease significantly, I knew it was bad. Not that I really understood in an intellectual sense but I knew it was not what I thought it would be. Then words, "Not functional for daily living skills," made my mind race out of control. What does that mean? Not fit for daily living? Not fit for daily living. Not fit for daily living? The words just raced around and around in my head. I kept turning them over and over trying to place a real meaning to them. Donna Lynn Brady mother of three career, masters school, goals, accomplishments is not fit for daily living. I died inside. My brain function plummeted I saw nothing, I felt nothing, I entered a deep darkness inside myself. I heard even less. All I could think about was not fit for daily living activities. What does this mean? Not fit means substandard like a piece of beef that is not fit to eat because it's spoiled. Daily living that means kids, school, work, husband, softball, eating, drinking, paying bills, driving, dishes, and cooking. Ok so I am a spoiled or bad person who is not allowed or deserving of school, work, kids, cooking, jobs, clearing. How could it be I had been doing all these things so well but I forgot, that was before the stroke.

Not fit for daily living. I looked at Christine. I said I have lost everything, She told me that I am now starting to realize what has happened to me. I said, "I have lost everything." Not everything she said, "Remember you still have your kids and family." At that moment those things she told me meant nothing. My heart and soul were empty.

After that session I went home. I don't remember how I got there whether it was by car, truck, bus or plane. I was sitting in my rocker. I rocked back and forth and back and forth without moving my eyes. My gaze was fixed the empty hole of nothingness that was my life. Nothing matters to me anymore. I couldn't feel anything for anybody not even myself. It was the windowpane that kept my eyes in focus, a focus of dark deep depression. A depression so deep that its hard to describe in words I had never heard or felt this way before. My entire being was swaying back and forth between life, between death, between reality and fiction. It was a movie that could not be real. I did not really understand what she was saying. I didn't want to, if I were allowed to understand what she said, all those words that were flooded my brain would have meaning. If meaning became a reality I would sneak back into a hole and never return. I dug a hole as fast as I could trying to get away from the reality that was chasing me. I was floating about the clouds now in a dream of bright sunshine where the games are being played. Strike on, I could hear as the figure swung at the first pitch. No, no, no never swing at the first pitch unless it's so perfect that not even a fly could be missed. Strike two the batter hit the bat to the ground to shake the demons that would let her connect to the ball away. I could hear the batter thinking to her self. Come on DJ you can do it! Don't mess this up! You have two runners on you get them in and Pudgy can drive you in. All you need is a hit a nice strong hit. No junk! Don't kill it. Relax just hit it with a nice level swing but hard. Watch the bat hit the ball. Check the pitcher's feet to read her throw. She's afraid of you DJ she doesn't want to pitch to you but she wants to pitch to Pudgy even less. Pudgy will hit me. The pitcher knows that but I just have to do my job first. The wind up, it's a rise! A rise ball, ha ha! Sucker that's my best pitch high and inside. The bat comes across effortlessly. Her face grimes as the bat cracks the ball. It's gone up up and away. It's going! Wow great hit I thought as she rounded third base! Her coach pats her back and gives her a high five. Come on Pudgy drive me in! As the girl turned to get the coach's signal for a hit and run I got a glimpse of her face, it was me. Her face turned to a drawn empty look like a face of death. How could it be? How could that be me? How could that vibrant person trying and wanting to make a difference be me? Today I am less, less of a person than she is. I am not really a person at all. I'm now only half of a person maybe even less. What makes you fit? What part of you is the part in combination with other parts that make's you fit for living? Is it your hopes, your dreams, your abilities, or your physical or mental presence? Is it your ability to read, write and remember? Today it seems it's all of them. I thought that I my life was worth and worthy of being as long as I could contribute to it in some way no matter how big or small. I'm not so sure now. Seems that they have standards for everything. What does normal, unnormal and subnormal really mean? I guess subnormal would be me. Not fit for living. How cruel to tell someone they are not fit to function of function will enough to be fit to live. He must have been day dreaming when he did the tests. He couldn't nor wouldn't say that about me. Maybe he forgot my vision problem. That is it the test results are someone else's. These things happen. Test results get mixed up some times.

As I sink further into my self I am periodically brought back up to the surface by Mike trying to hand me the baby. Donna here's her bottle she's hungry. I sit there in a mechanical exchange of motions not volunteering at all. Feed her, burp her, feed her, burp her, feed her burp her. I exchange no warmth of passion with her at this moment. Not because I don't want to but because I have no passion left. She would be better off had I died. Why did that priest pray to save my life? Had he known what they would say? Surly not for God is a kind God. He wouldn't play such a bad joke on me would he?

Monday strolled in front of me. Its time to go back to therapy. So what devastation is in store for me today? What will I lean today? My new word is dysfunctional and not fit. Ok lets go. I can barely even get myself to the car, buckle myself up, and sit for what seems an eternity to get there. Here we go. One flight, two flights, three flights to doom. Understanding was my enemy now. As the elevator door popped open I realized that this time when I swung the bat I missed and lost the game. Only this game was a game of life. As I push the heavy wooden office door open I try to fake a smile only nothing comes out. There are no words I am longing to say anymore.

I sit down in my chair as I always do. She opens the books, gets the pencils, she glances at me for just a moment. No words are in my brain there is pure emptiness. This is not like me and she recognizes that. I usually love coming to talk to her. I try to say how are you but that isn't even in my vocabulary today. As she settles down she said, "Your depressed aren't you." I don't know my response it wasn't much. That whole day is a blur. I don't recall what I said nor what she said. I do know that she made me feel a little better. She always did. For that wasn't the day that was chosen to hurt my brain even more.

The Fight

They can't seem to agree on where I am or where I should be. They seem to be fighting over me. When do I go home how long do I stay? How do you feel Ms. Brady, fine I reply. Why wouldn't I be fine they kept me so dopped on morphine that I slept all day. Without it my head hurt bad, with it my stomached hurt even worse. There are no choices for me. You keep telling me what it is I am to do. That I will recover. Recover from what? Why don't you talk to me not about me like I am not here. Who are you? Why does this CT/MRI tell you? What does that have to do with me? What did Mike say tell me? He told me I had a stroke. Ok I had a stroke it's over done with now let me go home to be with my kids. This happened after Amber right? How come it was only a neurological event then or a complicated migraine but now it is a stroke and you won't let me leave? Stroke what does that really mean. Ok I have a label for it now so let me go already. It will not be the first or last label I receive. What I didn't understand was that the label I world get now would be one I couldn't handle. I would learn that my new labels were going to be words like dysfunctional, depressed, suicidal, alexia, angry, hurt, and panicked. I would have to learn how to live with and accept some of these labels. Once a label is placed on you the glue that it used is like a piece of packing tape that rips the box each time you tug at it tying to get it off. With each tear comes a piece of your heart, accomplishments, and confidence. It takes years of hard work to rebuild the tears. If takes the ability to melt the box and then reform it into something useful again only this time since it's a recycled life and personality it isn't ever quite the same again. It can be whole, fruitful, purposeful, energetic, loving, have zest for life, but it will never be the same as it's original container.

The Cold

As the crest of the new fallen snow makes it's way to my toes, I am anxious, for when the coldness seeps so deep I can not feel it taking a part of me.

As I fight to keep the chill from reaching my heart I find that I can not control it. To lose control of your thoughts and emotions is to lose control of your existence.

For each time the chill of an uncaring soul touches my heart its like that snow that just slowly consumes your warmth, so does your heart chill in the night.

So when the chill sets in we fight even harder to warm ourselves, to do those things that make us feel warm before the stroke. To get back a moment of when the sun shown down on my head and warmed me. When this happens so too is my spirit warmed.

To fight each day to live, to fight each day to survive, to fight to keep my soul warm, so that the coldness of this earth does not consume us.

Hope

Matter of Existence
March 9, 1998

If you believe that energy as a single matter of existence carries life, that it can not be housed or truly controlled. If for one moment in time pure energy becomes the life force that swallows our soul, then you must also believe that God's prophesy of everlasting life has already been fulfilled. For if pure energy is what feeds the soul then we know that at that moment that precious second where life ends, the energy in it's quest to survive must find a new human soul. Is it possible that the energy of one can jump to another and live deep within its womb? That at that point when one life decides to end, it rests not within the soul of one already born but in its womb waiting until it's time to once again be reborn and feed the soul of another. To lay dormant as a spirit guarding against evil so that it can once again fly in the heavens. It must be at that precious point in time, clearly that second when the baby's head crests from its place of rest that the energy finds its way back to the unconscious of another. For if this survives in us all then each one of us has a guardian angel to help protect us and be our conscious. It is only a stroke of luck that the enkindled spirit of the energy through its lose is once again reborn. So take heed that we all have eternal life for it is in God's plan. It is only by chance that we are allowed to fully understand before it is our time to see.

To: Cain and Able Stroke Group

Hello again. I would like to take this opportunity to express my appreciation and "thanks" for letting me speak at your "Cane and Able" meeting this past week. You were all so very nice to me and I do appreciate that. I can only hope that the work audiences I speak to in September treat me as well.

I really enjoyed hearing your thoughts and your stories. You are the first group of survivors that I have met face to face. Too bad that I didn't take advantage of the opportunity to meet you earlier. Christine tried to get me to go the meetings but one thing I didn't lose was that stubborn streak in me. I think that I lost there for when I met you and talked with you, I realized that I missed out meeting and learning from a great group of people. Now I know.

Several of you asked me to come to your meetings and to join your group. I will come again, that I promise.

Thank you again. Take Care and May you each be blessed with all that is good in this life.

The First Time
June 25, 1998

She handed me the flyer the first time. I discarded it. She handed me a flyer the second time. I discarded it. Another handed it to me yet a third time. I discarded it. It was not until the last time that I learned that I shouldn't have discarded it the first time.

Healing hope

It is now that I know that there is hope in stroke recovery. That we each have lost but then we gain. The losses teach us what we can do physically and cognitively but the hope that we gain when we do something for the first time reaffirms our presence on this earth. I had no hope when I first had my stroke because I had no understanding of how things had changed for me. I then had despair over what I had lost and could not get back. Hope did not touch me until I started to talk to other survivors. Talking with other stroke survivors gave me the ability to see and feel their energy and presence. I could share my story and hear their stories. Each one of us keeps getting better. Hope is a forever thing it does not vanish in one day. I can say that we never know how much we can regain because we are changing our entire lives. As we change so do our abilities. Stroke may take from us but it can also give back if you let it.

We are the only ones that have had the opportunity to live two distinct lives. We have a chose to make ourselves better based on our past or we can choose to make ourselves wallow in our own despair. I think that I am lucky because I know whom those people are that I can count on in time of need. I know who my friends and family really are. Most don't get the opportunities that we have had since when they die it is often to late. I think about how much I have gotten when compared to what I have lost. Yes I have lost but in retrospect I have gained intellectually and spiritually more than I would have had this not happened to me. I have touched and been touched. I see without my eyes now but with my heart and a clearer sense of understanding of who I am and why. I have peace and comfort with less than what I had before. It has taught me that there is always hope for love and life no matter how bad it may seem. It is up to us each individually to look to the stars and touch one.

Chapter 4: Relearning

Work Day 1

Today is the day that I test all I have learned and all that I have felt. I see Christine at 9AM and then go to work. I am so afraid of what will happen if I mess I up? How will they react? What will they say? What will I say? I can't do this. I am sitting here at home waiting to go to therapy. Maybe I should wait. Maybe I am not ready. Christine.'s not really sure if I am ready either but I told her I had to do this. She told me it will be hard. It's my decision I said and now I am afraid I made the wrong one. I tried to eat but threw it up. I tried to drink but it wouldn't go down. Take a deep breadth it will be ok. I am driving to therapy and all I can see is nothing. All I feel is panic. I told her I am nervous she told me you'll be OK. I believed her. Through all of this she was always honest with me she did not make false promises or give me false expectations. I'm so glad I have one person who will be up front with me about my abilities.

Boy how fast this 50-minute session went. The days you want it to last forever it goes like a shot. I said goodbye and see you Wednesday. I made the choice to go back to work early because I didn't want return to work after therapy had ended. Christine could help me when I had problems at work. Unwittingly I didn't realize that my problems were increasing with my return to work. For months I could rest when I needed, think when I wanted to, eat when I was hungry, or be depressed when it hurt me. It was different now. I had to act and be normal. I couldn't let them see how bad it all really was. I got to work and everyone was great. I would only be working for four hours a day and I thought then that would only last for a few weeks not months. They were so kind to me. They hugged

When I Learn . . .Surviving Stroke with Pride

me, cried with me and made me feel good that I was back. They offered their help and support.

My boss even offered to read my mail to me. I was up front with them and told them what my deficits were so they were prepared when I came back to work. I thought that in my case being up front with them about what happened and my problems would make it easier. I am glad I did that because when I did make a mistake it wouldn't be a big surprise to them. They gave me six months to see if I could handle it. They were worried that I was coming back early but when I explained that Christine could help me reorganize my work day to make it as efficient as possible they understood. They were great. I am so very lucky to have been working for them when all this happened. My supervisors supported me through all of this and never belittled me when I would make a mistake. It's ok Donna you're doing fine don't worry about it, you've only been back a few weeks. They kept telling me that I was being to hard on myself.

That first day was filled with emotion and getting new passwords for my PC as I didn't remember my old ones. I didn't do much that day just talked and got reacquainted with the routine again. I was exhausted that day emotionally and physically. I don't remember my job being this tiring. I remember how easy my job was and looked forward to doing it again. I loved my job. Christine warned me that it would be different this time. It will be harder than it was before, a lot harder. I told myself it can't be that much harder because it was so easy before and I had been doing it for so long. Well I was wrong and she was right once again. She always had an uncanny way of telling me what would happen then letting me find out for myself. She always warned me but so often I wouldn't listen. Doesn't she hate being right so much? The first day was easy and I was exhausted after four hours but it was easy and I felt good. It was easy because I didn't work. They gave me a day to get aquatinted with everyone again so all I really did was talk with old friends.

In order to ease me back in they only gave me one of my programs back. I thought it was very nice and understanding of them. After several weeks I was beginning to realize just how hard it was going to be. I was unsure of each task I tried to do. It took me so long that I hated looking at my mail. I didn't understand things anymore I couldn't remember how to do them. I despised getting tasters. Work now frightened me. I panicked each time I was asked a question and thought I would die because my heart pumped so hard when I turned something in.

My savior came from a friend who I would learn has been the reason I can now do my job. I am not as detailed as I once was but her patience and care has provided me with the knowledge I needed to learn to survive at work. Karen would be my life force for survival during the week. Christine gave me ways to organize my new life at work but Karen gave me the confidence and retrained me to function there. She would proof my work help me find words and get me out of my panic attaches. She provided a sold foundation I depended on to succeed. With her guidance and my supervisors understanding I was allowed to have mishaps and learn from them. My success at work is a culmination of hard work, the tools that Christine gave me and the knowledge and support that Karen gave me. Mike provided the hugs when I was at the brink of breaking.

There have been a lot of great things happen at work but there has also been some bad. I have learned that stroke may bring some friends closer but drive others away. I remember a day, a specific day, it was sunny outside warm enough that I didn't wear a coat. I did not know that that day, which I thought was a normal day, would be one that almost drove me to the brink of death. It started out just like any other day. I got up got dressed and went to work. Little did I know within minutes from my arrival that someone who I had considered a friend would betray me, would once again turn on me. She took pride in my deficits and pointing them out to everyone at the top of her lungs. She said things like you can't read, I don't believe you, you don't do anything all day. You can't do it. She told me I was doing nothing not pulling my weight and that I would get her fired. I attributed her initial outburst to stress in her family life until today. Today, it was a Monday I remember that well. Two of my other team members had just arrived and were settling down to their desks. With a cup of coffee in my hand I went over to say hello as I always do. The conversation was light reiterating what our evenings had given us. For me it was the baby and girls and for them it was their pets. It was then that my ex-friend came up to us with a scowled look on her face. All I said was good morning, hope you had a good weekend, I told her I looked at a particular document and that it was fine with me. She blew, she hit me so hard and so fast that my head starting swimming my emotions form anger, to crying to panic, to dying. What was she doing what did I do. Did I forget something as she kept yelling and telling everyone that I couldn't read, that I couldn't do my job, that I was basically not fit for life. I was a damaged person in her eyes. "Yeah right you read them, I don't believe you, you can't read," she kept saying. You can't do anything anymore. You do nothing all day but talk. This went on for what seemed to be an eternity to me. I couldn't get out. I was standing between my teammates. No way out. Where can I go what can I do? I have to get out of here! I have to escape this terror! God get me out of here! What am I going to do? Why is she doing this to me. I could not go anywhere. Why was she doing this? I didn't disserve this. I thought she was my friend. I know now she isn't and never really was. Friends don't treat friends that way. If there was a problem she could have just talked to me about it. I looked at my team members they turned their heads and lowered them to their paperwork. I was devastated. I should have never come to work. Why did I think that I was ready? I couldn't handle anything that happened. I should have never tried. This was a big mistake I have to get out of here. I need to get away. Where are my keys damn it where are they? As the tears stared to well up in my eye's I just ran. I ran out the door and down the stairs as fast as I could. Four flights of stairs and out the door. I don't even know how I could make that now for I couldn't even see that well in the dark stairwell. I walked for a long time it had to have been at least an hour. I couldn't go back there. What if she was there waiting for me to pounce on me again. I can't do that again. I froze as I remember I had ran out so quickly that I had left my purse and my car keys at my desk. I was so afraid to get them. I turned and went to see Sue. Sue would help me she would know what to do. I had no phone. I could call Christine she would have an idea. I kept telling myself, "Donna she can't get you out of everything." She told you were going back too early. I made it to the second floor of Sue's building two buildings away from mine. It was like God put her there to wait for me. Sue was standing in front of me as I opened the door to the second floor. She looked at me and I collapsed on her shoulder. I can't do this. I can't do this anymore. I was in tears and trembling terribly. She got me calmed down she got it out of me what my ex-friend had done, another on of my friends had walked up and was ready to take care of the situation herself. What am I going to do? I have to work with her. Why would she do that to me? They were angry and I was defeated.

If was not the first time this intense feeling of hatred and helplessness had come over me. After regaining my composure I went back to my office. My teammates asked me if I was ok I told them I was fine. I told my boss what happened and left it at that. Months later they would realize that I was not over reacting to what happened as this same person showed her true colors to someone else. Eventually I would not have to work directly with her and I was relived. My life needs to be simple and I don't handle people being angry with me very well. For quite some time I thought I must deserve this treatment otherwise they wouldn't do this too me. It took me awhile to learn that my deficits should not to be used an excuse for someone else to be cruel. I am starting to learn very slowly that people are not as tolerant as they should be with others with disabilities or limitations. Limitation or no limitations we should all accept others as they are and support each other in the best way we can. I would find my work life would get easier as time went on. I learned that those who don't understand stroke and those who don't wish to understand use us to try to build him or her up. Anyone that must promote the misfortunes of another to make himself or herself feel worth while must have a very sad unfulfilling life. We can all learn from each other. I learned from that experience that sometime people are to scared to really understand. Now I do see this person at timed and I have talked to her. I am not angry with her anymore because that type of anger does nothing for me as a person. I may never understand why that happened but I think that when others are forced to face their own pain they get scared and react in ways that we would not expect. If everyone could truly understand they would admire our strengths and accomplishments no matter how small they may seem to be.

July 31, 1998

A memory came back today in the shower. I was freezing and thought a warm shower would make me feel better. I remember I was too weak to stand and the light that peeked through the keyhole pierced my brain. I sat as close to being under the faucet as I could so that the water would warm me. As I sat there with my legs pulled to my chest and my hands holding my head I wondered when the pain would stop. The gentle trickle of water seemed to pound against my head like a jackhammer trying to break through cement. Now I am in a place a bed with people running around me. I just kept praying that the pain would go away. It seemed that there was no end to the pain. As I lay in the hospital bed with tears from what seems to be every crevice of my body it was announced that I wouldn't receive a shower but a bath. I didn't know that when your in ICU you don't get to take showers your bathed by someone. As an unknowing victim who walks into a dark alley the figure of a person came into the room. It was the face of a man and that is all I could think try to ask what he was doing the words just flooded around in my head never reaching my lips. He brightened the room and it hurt my head. My brain was screaming what are you doing? You are not my husband! As he turned me from side to side the humiliation of just having a baby and the bleeding that follows hammered my conscious. He said to scoot your bottom as he placed a fresh pad under my female parts. He seemed to discount that these parts belong to me, a person, a female person whom has just brought life into this world. Am I just a body to be cleaned like you clean an animal with no care for the spirit that lies beneath the heart and head? It may be just a part of the job and it may feel normal to you but it is not normal to me. I am a self-conscious shy body and when you decided to send a male to bath me you hurt me mentally. I may not be able to communicate well but I am still me inside. It is wrong to assume that stroke takes my physical cares and dignities away. The stroke did not make me less deserving of the right to decide who could bath me. If I was in a coma I may not care but when I can open my eyes then you have to know that I can feel. You should ask yourself, if it was my wife, sister or mother would I want the same for them? My body is all I have after stroke why would you want to try to take that from me too. I know it was not out of cruelty but its hard when I lay there not to know why you made a decision and that didn't include me. Please just ask and if I care I will tell you somehow.

Needle in a haystack

The art of trying to relearn is a process of finding a needle in a haystack. Some stakes are big yet some are small yet it is that single needle that provides the tool we need to mend ourselves. It gives us the ability to fix what has been broken.

I remember a day in particular where I just couldn't understand. I looked at Christine with blank eyes. Eyes that told her that I it meant nothing to me. Three plus three she said. I repeated her words. Ok three plus three. Three what, three minutes or three hours? No Donna it's addition. She said, You need to take the numbers and add them together. I could not, did not, nor want, to understand. I was pretty good at math until the stroke. I made A's in my graduate classes in statistics and algebra. It was very disheartening to learn and fully understand that those thousands of dollars in post-graduate education just seemed to vanish into one plus one is two. I know that one plus one is two. Three plus there is? One, two, three, how do I add? What is adding? Another deficit, another problem and just one more thing I couldn't do.

I really learned to despise math it was hard. It still is. I didn't understand it nor could I really find a good use for it. I remember getting homework in math just to realize that my second grader had homework harder. It takes a certain amount of courage for a normal person to ask their second grader to explain basic addition. Imagine what it's like for those of us who were once good in math but had each ounce of confidence and abilities destroyed by the stroke. I need to learn to use a calculator that's it. I would only learn to use a calculator out of necessity not out of willingness.

Donna Brady

I remember learning numbers. I had been in therapy for probably a month. I wanted to call my boss at work. Now what possess a person who can't speak well to call their boss, the one responsible for their paycheck? I still haven't figured that one out yet (smile). I didn't have a clue not an ounce of thought that I shouldn't call until I tried to dial the phone. However that would stop me.

I picked up the receiver and looked at it. I could see the numbers if I held the phone to my left side as my right side had been damaged by the stroke. Ok, now what was my phone number? I remember 574. Ok I can call any 574 number and they could connect me. Now I tried to look in my phone book but that was pointless because I couldn't read. Ok, 574, 574, 574, 574, I stared at the phone. 5 ok where is the number 5. I couldn't see it. Damn my vision. I looked all around. 5 concentrate Donna you've had this number for years. I couldn't find it realizing this made my chest hurt. Oh my God I don't know how to dial a phone, what's wrong with me? It must be my vision either that or the number 5 is rubbed off of the phone. Even then I didn't get the point that math is a very normal critical part of life. I had to learn math to survive.

April hon come here please. Can you dial the phone for me? Sure mom what's the number? I think it is 574 something. Now mom that's not enough numbers she counted our number on her hand and said you need four more numbers. I told her just to pick some. In her young voice she said, Mom that doesn't make sense. I know that but I can't remember the number.

The phone rang and then an unfamiliar voice came on. This is Joe can I help you? Hi, my name is Donna Brady, I work for Connie I don't have her number. Can you find it and dial it for me because I had a stroke. Can you look up her number and connect me? He asked, "Is this for real?"Yes the voice on the other end said, ok you can look up my name if you want. Oh no this is weird enough that I

When I Learn . . .Surviving Stroke with Pride

believe you. Ms. Connie isn't answering her phone. Can you try Karen? Ok, the phone rang a voice at the other end said you've reached Karen may I help you? I repeated her name. Karen, this is Donna. I sense the hesitation in her voice. Hi Donna how are you? I fine you? Good I am doing well. I tried to chat but I still was having such a hard time talking. I could tell that it was all she could do to talk to me. I felt her heart sink as I tried to talk to her. The conversation was short. I didn't know it then but Karen would be the one that saves my sanity and helps me integrate back into work. I will always be grateful to her for her kindness. She has been on of the single most reasons why I was able to keep and progress in my job. Therapy ended but Karen stuck by me day in and day out. She let me cry. She lets me get mad, she just lets me be the new me. She doesn't ask for anything in return ever. She has always given me her time even when she has non.

She checked my work and tried to help me heal the wounds placed by the stroke. I wish that I would have known that she would be the one, the unsung hero and friend. Two souls that crossed and never let go. I still see Karen but not as much now. I am in a different area but when I am in her building I always try to take a moment just to giver her a hug and say hi.

Step by Step

It seems that each day brought something new something once understood but now lost. I didn't realize that my days had new meanings. Monday was the worst day because it was a weekly reminder that I was not healed and had so far to go. I welcomed Wednesday because the Monday fog of depression had diminished to a faint reflection. Friday seemed to whirl around me like the wind does before the storm. It took me quite some time to understand that I was going through a roller coaster of depression. Up and down and down and up my emotions would carelessly flow in and out of my day. I focused so heavily on the fact that Monday would so be here that I couldn't see the progress the other days provided.

I can't recall what event caused my brain to realize the gifts I had been given but at the point when I discovered some intellectual understanding of what had happened to my brain, my perception of what these three days offered also changed. Monday became a good day. I looked toward to sharing and learning from someone who only knew me as a stroke patient not the person from the life that had been so abruptly taken away. Wednesday's I shared my Monday's work with my children and husband and worked feverishly on getting all my Wednesday assignments finishing.. Only having one day between Monday and Wednesday helped. Each day step by step, day by day and hour by hour that is how I survived. Friday's became my bad days because there were two days between in which depression and craving for my old skills would haunt me. Friends and family ache for my previous self but unbeknownst to me that person ceased to exist mentally and physically.

So as I look back on Monday's, Wednesday's and Friday's they provided to be a step by step survival guide. Each day was representing a day to fight my way back to me. I tried desperately to grab a part of my lost capabilities. I was able to get through using each day as a stepping stone to the next. Each day lived was one day past, each day past was one day I didn't have to relive again. I began slowly looking forward to learning and trying to remember. It became my goal, my only single goal. Just like the little engine that could, I only had a single glimmer of what may lay ahead. That single glimmer slowly turned to a small sparkle. With each day leaned, whether it be Monday, Wednesday or Friday that sparkle started to develop into hope. The hope may have only lasted a second here and there but that too expanded to minutes, hours and then days.

So now that I have hope and I have understanding, I have and continue to develop the person I am to be. The new person inside of me is a conglomeration of who I was before in personality and who I am now is skills. Step by step, day by day, week by week and year by year that is how life is to be for me.

Chapter 5: From My Husbands Perspective

I consider myself a normal type of guy living a normal existence. A home, wife, three children, with Donna and myself holding down separate jobs in middle suburbia. Most of our free time is spent attending to the many needs and nuances of our young children. Our dreams are no different than most other families. Saving for our children's college education is one priority, while building our nest egg for when Donna and I retire being another, and when time and finances being available, taking an occasional vacation. Following a mundane yet not entirely uneventful or unhappy routine of school for the children, homework, chores and other curricular activities, these are the rules of the roost in our small yet happy household.

The birth of our three children being the pinnacle of our happiness, the consummation of our marriage and the closeness of family strengthened our resolve to fight and overcome a significant traumatic event which would attempt to cripple our small family, yet did not bury us in self-pity or remorsefulness, but allowed us to fight the battle of survival for an unforgiving and challenging event of loss in our lives.

Life is filled with many events that pull our families in different directions. Fate plays its role in our lives, which is sometimes controllable, and at other times can be very chaotic and unpredictable. I mention this because it was fate that brought Donna and I together.

It wasn't so far in the past when I watched Donna walk up the aisle at our church, beautiful, full of life, filled with the promise of our future life together. Dressed in a silky white satin gown, glowing in the radiance of all our future hopes and dreams. My emotions were extremely high that day, and I couldn't put any particular thought in my mind to keep me from shouting in blissful ecstasy, or in crying vainful tears. She had actually picked me to be that person that would share her life. The love that I felt for her that day was a very unique love, a free love. Free of all future hardships. Free of all worries and pressures of day to day happenstance. The world stopped that day, and everything up to that point of time would be our past life, and as we walked back down the aisle hand in hand, bonded by matrimony, becoming our new life together. In front of us laid all of our dreams for happiness, and our dreams of togetherness. The dreams of family, wealth, romance, and curiosity into what our new lives together would bring. A pure love which would continue to grow, inspired by our love and devotion for each other, so deeply rooted in our 15 years together, and yet, starting on that beautiful day when our free love intermingled, creating the start of the family which Donna and I are able to enjoy today.

The birth of our third child was, and still is a very memorable event. Everything proceeded so normally and smoothly during that time that there was no warning of what would happen next. Donna, and of course the rest of the family were all making the necessary adjustments of adding another beautiful child into our household. This particular day was as normal as any other day. We entertained friends and family, showing off our newborn to all those who came to visit. That evening, Donna developed a headache, which seemed to increase in intensity as the night wore on. She told me that she was going to take a shower to help ease the pressure inside of her skull. She often did this, as her past experience of running cool-water down the nape of her neck usually brought some relief from her headache. But this only aggravated her headache even more, and the intensity of pain increased to the point where she called my name. I'll never forget those next words that she spoke to me; "Mike, something's not right."

The next half-hour was a complete blur. I remember helping Donna out of the shower and assisting her in getting dressed. The pace was frantic as I called her mother to come watch the kids so that I could take Donna to the emergency room at the local hospital. She had to wrap a towel around her head as the lighting from inside of our home sensitized her eyes and increased the pressure and pain inside her skull. The ride in our vehicle on the way to the hospital was not the smoothest, and every small bump which jarred our vehicle sent deep moans of pain from Donna, always answered by my meek apology that I was doing the best that I could and that I was going as fast as I could. "Hold on Honey, we're almost there, hold on Honey, please hold on."

There was a very frustrating sequence of events which took hold of our lives and completely turned everything upside down. I could not have predicted the severity of the complications which would arise in the next hour and in the proceeding days. Every day became a new challenge for Donna as well as for our children and myself. We recognized that Time would be important to doing the things for which we endeavored, and now found time to be our greatest detriment. There is never enough Time.

I wheeled Donna into the Emergency Room on a wheelchair provided by their valet service and continued the process of signing her in. This process seemed to have lasted hours, but in actuality probably only lasted several minutes. During this time, Donna continued to hold onto the towel, which was wrapped around her head. In a brief conversation that I had with Donna at this time, she was able to tell me that her headache was extremely severe, "I have never had a headache this bad before." I stood next to Donna at this point, worrying if the pain that she was suffering would cause her to lose consciousness, causing her to fall out of the wheelchair and onto the floor. With the minutes seemingly turning into hours, panic started to set in. Here was my wife, my love, the mother of our three small children, rife with pain, and there wasn't anything I could do to help her, too comfort her. I was totally helpless as I watched the hospital personnel remove Donna from her wheelchair and laid her on the gurney. Someone told me that they were taking her to have a Cat-Scan performed and that I would be notified after this procedure was completed. I sat down in the emergency sitting room and waited. Totally lost in worry and thought, I couldn't even begin to know how long I actually sat there. It was when they announced my name that I came out of my self-imposed trance and followed several personnel down many aisles to a place where my wife was still prone on the gurney, seemingly in a deep sleep. This area that I now stood in seemed to be some sort of holding area, a nook off the last aisle that I approached before seeing my wife. Donna was surrounded by four or five people, all clad in white hospital garb. The nook was encircled by doors on three of its sides, all announcing the complicated machinery and equipment that they held beyond their closed doors. It was then that one of these people approached me. He introduced himself as the person in-charge of this department, and proceeded to tell me the results of Donna's Cat-Scan.

I prepared myself for the worst, but I was totally unprepared emotionally for what he would tell me next. He continued speaking to me in his medical jargon of what was causing Donna's condition. I nodded in acknowledgement as though I understood what he was telling me. "Donna is suffering from a subarachnoib hemorrhage." All wild eyed and attentive, I soaked in every word he spoke, as if we were holding this conversation in slow motion. "What did this mean? What was he saying?" Donna was suffering from an inter-cerebral bleed. She was bleeding, deep within her brain. "Was surgery an option?" Performing an operation of this kind by cutting open her cranium to try and stop the bleeding inside could cause more permanent injury to the brain than a more cautious and conservative approach of waiting for the vein to stop bleeding all by itself. It was also possible that the bleeding would not stop and a decision would have to be made later. The doctor and myself both agreed together that a wait and see attitude was our best option at this time, and that we would both hope and pray that the bleeding would stop on its own. Donna would be moved to the hospitals Intensive Care Unit in Serious condition, where she would be monitored 24 hours-a-day, until hopefully, the bleeding would stop on its own. It was then that I broke down .... and cried.

The ICU at this particular hospital was of a serene and peaceful nature, with none of the noises and distractions in which I normally associated with other places in this hospital. The staff on duty spoke in hushed whispers and were very attentive to the needs of Donna and also of myself. When I entered Donna's room, I was stunned to see all the wiring attached to her skull, the wires which protruded from under her gown, the I.V. tubes, and the catheter tube which extended from her person in a spaghetti like mass. The constant humming and beeping of all the surrounding monitoring equipment echoed in the stillness which was present all around me. Here was the woman I loved, prone in an almost comatose state, fighting for her very existence, her life. Thus would begin my vigil of sitting next to her bed, holding her hand and caressing her arm, the long hours turning into days, somehow trying to communicate to her that I was by her side, waiting for some kind of miracle that would tell me that this had been some kind of horrible mistake, and that when I woke up from this nightmare of a dream, she would be standing next to me, smiling and happy, radiant and loving.

Being aware that the lives of our three young children depended on my ability to remain strong for some sense of normalcy to reign at home, I needed to develop a strategy for them, for us, so that our household would not develop some sort of dysfunctional breakdown or would not be able

When I Learn . . .Surviving Stroke with Pride

to handle any crises for which I would be unprepared. We didn't need any additional adversities which could cause any number of severe repercussions in the minds of our small children. I spoke to the children the best way I knew how, explaining to them that their mother was suffering from a very bad headache. Because her headache was so bad, their mother would need to be taken care of at the hospital by a doctor, who would help their mommy get better. "She also told me to tell you that she loved you, and that she missed all of you, and that as soon as she could, she would come back home, and that she would give all of you a big hug."

Keeping any sense of normalcy at this time was highly improbable, yet not totally impossible. My days consisted of waking up with my children every morning in our own home. This was very important for me, and for my children, I am sure, and I would never deviate from this during the entire time of Donna's illness. I would feed the children their breakfast, and then drive the oldest to school every morning. Then grandma would arrive, and I would drive to the hospital and sit with Donna until mid-afternoon, and at which time, I would return home to pick up my child from school, and what little quality care that was available to me, spending it with my three young children. During these sessions, I would try to update them on their Mother's progress. I would also try to ease their anxieties and their precious little tears by telling them that their mommy was getting better every day, and that soon she would be coming home to join us. This was always followed by a group hug, and then dinner, which put a tremendous amount of pressure on me, as my culinary skills left a lot to be desired. Macaroni and cheese one day and hotdogs the next was an easy way out, however, my conscience would get the best of me, and I soon found myself experimenting on my children with many original and unoriginal concoctions. Of course, my children had the final say, and if I failed miserably, they let it be known in no uncertain terms that the meal that I tried to feed them was "yucky".

Of course, being the good father that I try to be, I would resort to my back-up plan which consisted of, "you guessed it", macaroni and cheese. This was then followed by bathtime and then preparing them for their travel and care at our friends home. After this, I would travel back to the hospital and spend the evening with my wife, always staying until she received her pain medication, which usually occurred between 10 and 11 o'clock at night. After assuring myself that she was able to rest peacefully, or what I had hoped would be a comfortable and uneventful slumber, I would leave to pick up my children and take them home, briefing them on their mother's status, reading them a bedtime story, and tucking them into bed for what I hoped would be a good night's rest. This left the end of my day to catch up on housework; laundry, dishes, cleaning, vacuuming, and other chores, which would need to be completed so as to make our home presentable in appearance and functional for the next day of activities. I learned by accident not to ignore any chore for too long without giving it my attention, as anything left unattended would accumulate unmercifully, and that my chores for the following day would be totally unforgiving.

During the time that I spent with Donna, I was able to learn more about the medical phrases and terminology's that were used by the medical staff at the hospital. Donna and I were befriended by an attending male nurse who worked one of the shifts in the Intensive-Care-Unit. He was kind enough to help me reach an understanding of what was really happening inside of Donna's brain. She had suffered a "Sinus Thrombosis," a clot in the brain which had blocked the flow of blood through her brain, and which in turn caused a blood vessel to rupture, precursor to a "Subarachnoid Hemmorhage", a bleed within her skull. This in-turn induced a "Hematoma Bruise," a collection of blood which accumulated around the injury, putting pressure on all parts of the brain-tissue that came in contact with the bleed. The bruising would cause scar-tissue to develop in this area, and would be a constant reminder to Donna, in all probability, lasting for the rest of her life, as her proceeding headaches all seem to center at the very point of where the internal injury had occurred.

The second day at the hospital was when Donna and I had a visitor, a chaplain, who had come to see Donna and provide prayer and encouragement, a sort of last will and testament to God. This was a very emotional event for both Donna and myself. We held hands and recited the Lord's prayer, and then the chaplain took the lead in reciting another prayer asking God to bring his healing powers down upon Donna, so that "she may once again lay her eyes upon her children, and hold them in her arms." Even though Donna's communicative skills were greatly diminished, she did manage to tell the chaplain that "she was in a lot of pain and that she didn't want to be hurting her family anymore. She had made peace with god and she was now ready to die."

I then left the room not wanting Donna to see the tear's which were freely flowing down from my eyes. This was also an opportune time to let the Chaplain have a few private moments with my wife. When he left the room, I thanked him, and then reentered Donna's room to take up my customary position next to her bed. I held her hand, rubbing her arm in my usual manner, trying to bring her attention back to me. I did not know what she was thinking, but she did see the tears on my face, and then said to me, "I'm sorry honey." I told her that what had happened wasn't her fault. All I wanted was for her to get better. I then proceeded to tell her that it was too much of a burden for me to raise our three young girls by myself. They would need their mother, and that she would have to help me in taking care of their needs. I promised her that she would be no burden to any of us, and that it was important for her to get better, so that she could come back home, and that we would be a family again. When I left the hospital that night, on the way home to pick up my girls, I wept, wondering if I would ever see Donna alive again.

Donna would suffer from her intercranial-bleed for three days, and then just as suddenly as it had started, the bleeding stopped.

During the time that Donna was incapacitated in the hospital, it was important for me to stay focused on the challenges that lay before our family. Making sure that I was able to at least spend some time with my girls, being just one of the goals that I had set for myself. With the loss of their mother's attention now apparent to my young ones, I just couldn't pawn off all of my responsibilities as a father on someone else. Our children would need to have contact with me, as I was the only parent available at this time. They were also able to feel some closeness to their mother, through me, without actually seeing or touching her. My updates to my children about how their mother was doing, I think, became a critical part of their understanding of a situation in which they didn't really understand, yet trying too in the only way that their young minds would allow.

Our newborn child, nine days old when Donna experienced the beginning of her trauma, was a special little problem that would tax my inner strength to what I had thought were my very limits. This little precious joy of ours would in her own special way, communicate the many needs of changing her soiled diapers, satisfying her hunger pains, holding and coddling her, and providing any external stimulation that she so desired at times that were convenient for her, but brought me to the brink of exhaustion. Those small interludes of two to three hours that would provide me the small quantities of sleep that my mind and body craved for was simply not enough. It was during this time that the people that I would meet during our ordeal would comment on the fact that I looked tired, and that it didn't look like I was getting enough sleep. Then they would offer too help in any way that they could, in any way possible, which would allow me to get the rest that I desired. I will always remember those sincere suggestions of consideration, as they meant that there were people that cared for Donna, as well as myself and our children. Looking back now at these generous offers of support, I guess that I might have been a little bullheaded at the time, wanting to prove to myself that I was capable of handling this crisis, as there was no doubt in my mind that if this situation had been totally reversed, Donna would have been able to handle herself and our three children in a proud fashion. I was well aware of the fact that my energy levels were running dry, and that I was benefiting from the pure adrenaline that was running through my veins, but I would refuse to let anything hamper my ability to survive this crisis, with family intact.

With the separation of a loved one from our family, the uncertainties of our future, and the urgent and important crises which faced us every day, it was very important that I find the strength to continue to strive for the goals that I had put in front of me in my quest for family survival.

I found this inner strength in two very important thoughts that I still carry with me to this day. First, there was Donna, fighting the most important battle of survival, the fight for her very own life. I'd be dammed if I wasn't going to do my own part and fight my own battles with uncertainty, which weighed heavily upon my family, and at any time could throw my children and myself into an abyss of deep depression. By keeping the internal structure of my family surviving in a climate of our own uncertainties, we could best prepare ourselves for when we would greet Donna with open arms on the day she would eventually come home.

Secondly, I knew if I concentrated on keeping the stability of my family functioning as normally as possible during this crisis, and that God knew that I was doing my part, that he could concentrate on helping Donna to survive and overcome this critical part in our lives which threatened to destroy our family.

The day Donna came home from her extended stay at the hospital was a very joyous moment for our daughters and myself. It seemed at that time that our life would return to normal, and that I would finally receive the rest and normal routine, which I craved for more than anything else. Of course, only in children's books does the story end ith "happily ever after." The real battles were just beginning. Donna had suffered a terrible brain injury, which incapacitated her and left her with several deficits in her cognitive skills and memory. Fortunately, she did not suffer any paralysis or any long term muscle incapacity. Because of her injury, she was very weak physically and would require a wheel chair during her recovery. Donna saw that wheelchair as her enemy and treated it with disgust, finally pushing it aside one day and letting everyone know that she would not be using it any more. The wheelchair became a painful reminder that something terrible had happened to her and because of this, her first goal of recovery and independence that she yearned for was the elimination of that painful reminder. Donna then determined that driving to her own therapy sessions was her next step. This was no small achievement on her own part not because she had to learn how to drive again, but she now had to deal with the loss of her right side peripheral vision which was damaged and taken away by her stroke.

Some of her deficits were explained to us from the medical staff, but others were discovered purely by accident. One day I walked into the kitchen to discover that Donna was crying. I asked her what was wrong and she told me that "I know that thing on the wall is important and I can see the numbers, but I don't know what it's supposed to tell me." She was talking about the clock and she couldn't tell what time it was. Another deficit that she suffered was her ability to read. Because of this, she was unable to help her daughter with her homework and unable to read books for her children. This sent her into a downward spiral of depression. Things became worse, as she became more aware of how much the stroke had taken from her, the things that she had taken for granted and, the ability to function normally were gone.

Though I did my best to help during her recovery, providing her with my love and compassion, I knew it wasn't enough, as I fully didn't understand what was going on in her mind. Then one evening I entered the kitchen only to find Donna slamming her fists into the sides of her temples, crying out that she hated herself. She hated what the stroke had done to her and what it had taken away from her. She felt lost with feelings' of hopelessness and the desire to end her suffering. I grabbed her arms and then I embraced her. She was crying, and when I asked her what was wrong, she told me that she "felt helpless and that she felt that she was a burden upon our family and that she wished that she was dead." This was the second time that she had mentioned those words to me.

We decided then that Donna would use her energies to pursue the help that she needed and that I would take care of everything else. This decision allowed her to focus more on her recovery and to give her the time she needed to seek the answers for which she seemed determined to find. "I'm not going to let this thing beat me Mike," she told me. "I'm going to get better." she said. At times, her recovery would make tremendous strides, and on other days, no sign of healing would be noticed. There were good days and bad days, days where Donna was able to regain some semblance of the past, and there were bad days when Donna was to discover that something had been lost, taking away a part of her. Being able to accept what had happened to her, I think, was one of Donna's greatest strengths, which I think helped her to bury some of the demons that tormented her. Recovery and healing from her injury will last Donna's lifetime. That is what we have been told. But now at least, time is on our side.

It was a cold day during the late stages of winter with ice and snow everywhere. The sun was shining fiercely and the steam from our breaths seemingly lingered in the cold frigid air. I pushed Donna in her wheelchair from her therapy session up to our vehicle, which was waiting for us in the valet section of the hospital. As the valet opened up the passenger door of our vehicle, we both then made an attempt to help Donna to remove herself from the wheelchair into the passenger seat. She told us, "I don't need any help." The valet looked at me but I just shrugged my shoulders. On our way back home I looked at Donna wondering what was going on in her mind. She looked at me and said, "I know I'm not a victim Mike. I just found out today that I am a SURVIVOR." As I drove home I couldn't help but smile. I always knew that Donna was a fighter, and now for some reason I knew that Donna was going to get better, that everything was going to be all right.

Chapter 6: How kids cope

How they react to the stress

I am sure that there are a lot of books that deal with the stress children experience during crisis. I am not a psychologist but a mother of three who watched and felt her children's pain at night as they lay in their beds unsure of where there mom had gone. When I first had the stroke my children were scarred. They thought I had died because I was no where to be seen and they were not allowed to see me in the intensive care unit. They were so positive that I had died that we made a tape of me while I was in the intensive care unit so they could see that I was still alive. That was a very hard tape to make in my condition; however, it is amazing what your spirit will help you accomplish when your children's well being are at stake. Mike had to help prompt me so I would sound ok when I tried to speak the words. My children watched that tape all the time and even now they like to watch it so they can see that I am better. My children internalized a lot of the grief, hurt and anger they felt over me being so sick. We would deal with the stomachaches and sleepless nights when I returned home. Mike and I would spend hours giving reassuring hugs and kisses and talking with them to help them understand that it's ok to be sad, mad, and ask questions about mommy and why she has changed so much.

When I finally came home they were even more frightened because of my fragility. I was not the same mom that left them just a few weeks earlier. They were only 7 and 5 years old. All they knew was that I had a baby and now I was sick. It took time for them to really understand that mommy was ok when she came home with the baby, it was not the baby's fault that mommy had gotten so sick. I really wanted the kids to understand that the baby did not cause me to get sick. I did not want them blaming their baby sister for what had happened to me. We talked about how they get sick sometimes after they play with friends but that it's not their friend's fault they are sick it's the tiny bug that made it to their tummy. I remember Amber, my 5 year old, would sleep next to me holding my hand. One night I asked her, "Why do you hold on so tight to mommy's hand when you sleep?" She said, "I am afraid you will die if I let go." I have learned that we often do not give children the credit they disserve for their understanding of how bad things can be. Our children are both fragile and strong at the same time.

I think the stroke was hardest on my oldest. She felt very betrayed at first as I could not help her with her homework nor did I understand her problems in school. Kids would sometimes teaser her. She became a very serious child early on having seen what illness can do to a person. She would often ask me if the same thing would happen to her. Her stomach would hurt from the pain she was feeling inside. That would get better with my reassurance that I was doing well and the more recovery she would see in me. I remember times that she would be so positive about how I was doing when I myself was not sure I would make it. With a big smile she would tell me how good I was doing since I couldn't do that before. She would ask me if I would be a 100%. I always told her yes. I did that not trying to give her false hopes but to reinforce that I was getting better. I was up front with her and she understand that I may not be able do all of those things I could before but being a 100% is being her mom and taking care of her and her sisters. For the health of my children I tried very hard not to let them see just how uncertain I was of my own recovery. Children need support. They need to know that their needs will be met no matter the circumstances that lay ahead. I find now that our definition of a child's need is not always what we as adults think it is.

It is often just what it should be love and stability. It is not all the "extra stuff" that we are told we must be able to give them. Children do not judge us by the "things" they judge us by our love and our ability to provide the basic necessities in life. Those necessities I now define as love, food, home, and pride.

So what did I learn from my children? I learned that I must fight for my children to heal from stroke. The struggle of stroke is not just mine it all that is affected by me. Stroke has a lasting effect on our children, family and life. My children are very compassionate. That compassion was taught through our pain. I may not have been able to teach them that had I not had the stroke so some good did come from all the bad. They have learned that we all have something to offer. My oldest has learned that a hug, "I love you" and a kiss can melt the pain of learning. We have all learned that what we offer should not be judged by the quantity of which it is offered but by the kindness of the heard that it is build and given.

Helping or children recover

I have learned that not only do I have to make a commitment to myself to recover but I must also commit to my children that I will help them to recover. I must help them learn when I learn. I don't know when I first realized that my kids were affected by the stroke. I should have but I was so focused on my own recovery that I lost sight of their recovery needs. I started very slowly with my kids. Not out of compassion for them but out of necessity so that I could keep up. I have learned the hard way that slowing down can provide what we need to help our children understand and recover too. I let them have a part in my relearning how to read, write and see. I let them ask questions about why I was so afraid all the time. I was truthful and up front with them. Kids know if you are lying. My kids often needed the reassurance that my own answers would not change. They were afraid that I would get worse instead of better or that I would have another stroke. It's ironic that our worries were often the same. There we a lot of very painful moments my children experienced during my recovery. I remember the pain in their eyes when they would ask me to help them with a word in their spelling book just to find out that I couldn't read. The majority of my recovery would take place in the first year or so following the stroke but what we have to remember is that it is the first few months that burn memories into their brains. I use to ask my kids what they remember of me when I first came home from the hospital and it amazes me to think that their memories are so vivid at the beginning but seem to fad as I recovered. I hate the fact that my kids would come home from school just to see me in so much pain from the headaches that I would basically turn into a zombie motionless and distant. As my brain tried to heal itself the headaches came in rounds as it bashed my brain against my skull. It was very hard to keep it emotionally together so that my kids didn't feel the brunt of the pain. We would work as a family trying to come to grips with the changes the stroke left for us.

My therapist suggested that I write my own thoughts down to help myself recover. I decided that my kids should do that also. For the 5-year-old that was hard we mainly just talked and hugged as she drew pictures of me in the hospital and in the wheelchair as they pushed me to therapy. My 7 year old really thought writing her own book about the stoke was a great idea. She was energized that she could be a published author. I think it gave her something to be proud of that related to my stoke. It gave her the ability to be proud that I had survived and that it was ok that I was not the same as I was before. April and I talked a lot about sharing the information she had learned with her friends at school so that they wouldn't be afraid of me. It was amazing how well she communicated her thoughts on paper and how

When I Learn . . .Surviving Stroke with Pride

distinctly she remembered the night I had the stroke and the events that followed. During the initial months I was like a kid myself so it was much easier for me to relate to her than to my own husband at times. I remember her talking about kid things and being somehow knowing that I shouldn't be so enamored with it because I was her mother not one of her school mates. April worked on her "book." Once the book was finished we had it published in the "New Hope" newsletter. April's "book" although not long in length is very rewarding to my family. I am including her thoughts here. They are her words I just typed them up for her.

Aprils Book: My mommy had a stroke.(by April Brady/age 7/1998)

Hi my name is April and I would like to tell you a story about my mom having a stroke. My mom had a terrible stroke she was really sick for three months. I was scared and our mom had to stay in a chair to rest. My mom had a baby girl named Alexa Cheyenne Brady. When my mom had the stroke she had it after Alexa was born. And Alexa is nine months old now. And she can walk with something to support her.

When my mom was in her bedroom all of a sudden my mom couldn't see with her glasses. And that's the beginning. My next door neighbor Vivian came to watch me and my two sisters until my grandma got home. All of us were very scared so was my grandma. My daddy took my mommy to the hospital. When daddy brought my mommy home my mommy couldn't talk the same. My mommy had to eat cold things because her head hurt a lot so we got to see her after school in her bedroom. And we got to bring food and drinks to her. My mom was proud of me April, Amber and Alexa. And when she had the light on her head hurted but now it doesn't hurt as much. My mom could only eat soft things because it hurt to chew and her head hurt when she ate hard things but now it doesn't hurt to chew anymore. When my dad took my mom to the hospital I was afraid that I'd never see mom again. But she did come back from the hospital so my mom is feeling much much more better.

Then my mom started to go to therapy. She had to roll into the elevator but we had to help mom and we had to roll her to the therapy room. And we had to wait for almost two and half hours but we only waited for one hour. And my mom's therapist name is Christine. And we called her Ms. Christine. My mom sat in this really small room only five people can fit in that room. Ms. Christine was really busy with my mom. Because she had to relearn how to write, and read all over again. And my mom got much much better. And now my mom goes to physical therapy. And me and my sister drew pictures but I colored a picture from our coloring book and I drew her one. My sister Amber drew two sheets of paper with five ballerinas on each sheet of paper. My mom had lots and lots and lots of homework. My mom is a hundred percent now!

So when I learn I see that the most precious gifts come in small packages. I see the sun and its rays and remember that even a bad day can be good. It is up to us to make that dark clouds of stroke turn in to shimmering rays of warmth and kindness.

Chapter 7: Write, Write, Write

Once I had started healing from the stroke I found that my mind was flooded with words that just needed to get out. I don't remember why the words started just that when they would come I had to make sure I wrote them down immediately. I kept a pen and paper next to my bed, in my purse, in my car and in my kitchen. I found that if I did not write the words down right then that they would be lost forever. I would often take pen and paper with me when I would shower because they often seemed to flood my senses when the warm water rushed down my back. My best words seem to come when I was lost for the verbal words to express what I was experiencing. I could often tell a story in my head but seems to never be able to express those same words in the manner in which I felt them. I really will never know if the words and thoughts I have are really mine. I often feel that they are just an expression of my brain trying to regain control of it surroundings.

I have learned that people love to express themselves verbally but often lack the tools to do so effectively. I have found that with all the pain I have suffered with the stroke I am more able to let people know when I am happy and when I am sad. I also find that I relate better to those who can share in difficult times. The writings that follow must be captured in heart. To merely read the words without reaching for their expression will leave you empty. To fully gain control of our consciousness we must feel each thought and live each word when we think it. The mere art of speech does not mean that we take the time to feel the words as they flood from our consciousness.

I have asked a few of my stroke recovery friends if getting over and dealing with the physical effects of stroke is harder than the cognitive ones. I was surprised at their answer. We all know that man is not merely a reflection of himself physically but a reflection of his heart and soul. Both these men who have very limited speech agreed that the hardest is no learning to walk again, lift their arm, clinch their fist or use their leg but to speak words at will. I can only relate from what I remember when I couldn't speak. I must admit that although my memories are very vivid in most instances now that I have my speech back I fight to remember how hard it was when I didn't. I do not want to lose that because I want to always remember those feelings so I can use them to help others.

I remember having the words flood my brain with no release. It is being trapped inside a prison called your brain. The only way out is through speech, reading and writing. Stroke takes those things but often leaves the memories of the former self to struggle against the one who has been left behind. It is like an episode of the X-Files. I am fortunate because I can now write, read and speak the words I need to get what I am asking for. I may not have the ability to use these words like I could in my former life but I have the ability to express myself at will, have it heard, have it responded to, and have it understood. I have learned that we often take the simple things like speech for granted. The ability to see, hear, and speak are life's more treasured pleasures it is therefore our duty to take care of them. It is speaking with them that I realize just how fortunate I am to have come so far.

One of my friends who is a stroke survivor amazes me at her own view of how people are. We try to meet for lunch every so often. I have seen people get visibly frustrated with her when she tries to give her order. It angers me greatly so see people treat her this way. Just because her speech does not fit their norm does not give them the right to speak to me directly when they should be speaking to her. Who are we to judge those that have so much to offer? Who are we to not show them the respect they have earned by their own recoveries? When I learn, I learn the most from those like me. I learn from them each time I see their smile and hear their laugh. We must make a good life for each person we touch. So when I learned from these three people I learned that I must write down what I think and share it with anyone who will read them so that I can may a difference for us all.

The following are writings that I have written since my stoke. The majority of them were to by best estimate around between the 1-2 years after stroke. People have asked me to share these with them and I have shared some on occasion. I did not write for pleasure before I had my stroke. I do this now since I have learned that I must treasure even the small things that I have been given since my stroke.

Clouds

It is the sky that I venture to for freedom. The soft billows of clouds that give us the ability to relax to feel for that moment that all our pressures are gone.

For when I fly into the heavens to see and touch a cloud it is the comfort of the freedom that it gives me. I think my life is like that cloud so high up into the sky for each day I look to it for comfort and direction.

A Child's Kiss

As I hold her and she places her soft warm cheek against mine. My heart fills with the warmth of a spring summer day and the scent of roses that touch the top of your nose. As I fill my lungs with air I can smell the gentle fragrance that gives you peace.

When your child places on her own the first kiss of love your soul remembers it. It takes your mind back to a place of comfort without compromise.

Donna Brady

Short thoughts

　　For when she placed that first love drawn kiss on my cheek I felt love. Love that only a child can give.
　　As the sun set over the mountain
　　The peace I had once loved,
　　　　Desperately fought to once again touch my heart.

As I recounted the blessings I have received,
I realized I have had more than my share.

If I have only learned one thing in this life,
　　it is that the power to touch and to be touched is
　　both good and bad.

She told me today that it would be OK and,
　　for the first time I believed it.

With each kiss I lay upon her small soft cheek,
　　I forgot about all the bad,
　　and for that moment my life is perfect,
　　once again.

I looked at my computer today,
　　and started to cry.

What a fool am I,
　　for so many can't even see.

I felt sorry for myself again,
　　wish I would stop,
　　feeling sorry for myself that is.

As he looked into my eyes,
　　I knew that the news was bad,
　　I wondered if I could take anymore.

I used one of her memories today,
>   the one when she said "you've come so far".

Another memory came back to me.
I use to be a good ball player,
>   I wonder what I am good at now.

Tomorrow is testing,
>   I am nervous.

I dread the results.
I don't know if I can handle it again.
I know I am a little better,
>   but still not good enough.

As I drove down the road,
>   I felt a sense of despair.

I know only on person who did not know me before,
>   and she will be gone soon.

I hate it when people just won't accept that I may not get much better.
I wonder who I will talk to when my sessions end.
I wish I was different than I am.
I care too much about people.

If life was so simple,
>   it would be to easy.

It's only the bad times that make the good feel so rewarding.

I feel a sense of piece when I draw upon a new memory.
I feel a sense of grief when I draw upon the old ones.

Eyes of presence,
>   eyes of presence show you who you are,
>   your heart any soul are revealed.

It's the ability to draw another closer,
    without them even understanding why.

Are you OK?
    My brain is failing me,
        is that OK?
    My back is failing me,
        is that OK?
    Others choose my path,
        is that OK?
    Life is failing me,
        is that OK?
    I pray God doesn't.

They say there is a light at the end of the tunnel,
If there is, then the path that I have chosen is winding,
    for I can't see the light.

If the light is at the end, at the same place death is,
I pray my path is twisted even more.
An angel came to help me, at first I didn't see her.
    Later after I did, it was too late for I had already lost her.
A second angel came to visit,
    this time I made sure she knew it.

As I watch my children play,
    I wonder will life ever be that simple again?
I guess it can't for our innocence is gone.

Happy is the mother that can gaze upon her children.
Sad is the mother that can't.
Death is the mother who has lost hers.

As I glance back,
    I remember where this life started,

As I walk through the door,
>   I forget about the old one.
As I look up into the sky,
>   I know I can live this new one.

Death, the art of dying.
It is not until you attempt death that you realize that it is an art.
It is not until you fail that even death is hard.
To hurt oneself is easy.
To survive is courageous.
Only the strong survive,
>   for death is the easy way out,
>   I think.

As I look over the calmed waters,
>   I remember when life was so simple.
As I sip that cup of coffee,
>   I relive that moment.
For when we have had piece in our lives,
>   we can always find our way back,
>   to piece.

As she pulled my neck I tried not to breath,
>   to hold the pain in so she could not see,
>   for seeing me is seeing pain,
>   and I don't wish pain on anyone.

It wasn't until I couldn't say anything that I realized,
>   I wasn't over it yet, the stroke took more of me than
>   I realized.

I thought that once I could read, write, and remember that others would not treat me different. I have now learned that people are cruel and the curliest don't want to understand.

Donna Brady

My stroke touched my daughter as school today,
As I wiped her tears,
    I told her that its OK to cry,
    but don't cry for me,
    cry for the boy who had to tease you because he didn't understand.

It was a angel that helped me heal.
It was a daughter that gave me the spirit to fight.
It wasn't until I was well that I realized my daughter was my "Angel".

As I read out loud, the pain in my heart grew,
    for I thought that silencing my voice would silence my pain.

Parents control the child's life,
    destiny and thoughts, too bad, we were all children at one time.
Depression, sacrifice, it is my life now.
Hope, smiles and hugs only pop in from time to time.

It is the meaning of life that we search for,
    it is the meaning of hope that we strive for,
    it is the meaning of piece that we all must find.

We are born trusting,
    we are taught not to.
A child love is unconditional,
    until its trust is broken.

I have learned more than most and less than some.
Those who taught me the most I hold deep in my heart.
Those who taught me the least I don't.

My heart, body, and soul are yours Lord,
  I was born from you and will return to you,
  please let me nourish the heart, body, and soul
  of those you have blessed me with to raise for you.

It wasn't until the dark of night that the sun's light descended upon my spirit. It was the darkness that lifted my spirit to a height that I never thought I would see again. As the sun crested the top of the highest mountain, so did my spirit. It was then I found peace and tranquility.

The Fight
It was not until I fought to get my way back to me that I realized my fight had only begun.

To speak a word and have it not heard, to think a thought and have it mean nothing, to write a letter and have it be empty, that is the way the fight begins.

The "me" in me is no longer normal.

To work each day on survival, to measure your accomplishments by inches, that is how we survive. That is how the fights begins and ends.

To have a stroke is easy, to survive a stroke is hard.

To fight your way back to who you were is impossible for once stroke touches your life, your life is changed forever.

The fight does not stop until the you, you once knew is a distant memory, and the new you has immerged. So help us find the new "me" for now the old one is a distant reminder of who we used to be.

As he placed her small soft body against mine the warmth of her spirit nested again my soul. As she dug her pale little nose, that smelled of a splash of a gentle drop of rain water unto my neck, it was then that my heart understood that this was the purpose of life.

Donna Brady

Reflections Feb. 20, 1998

As I look back on all I have done and all I have experienced, I know that it is how we reflect on our selves that guides us along the way. Its how the wind whispers in our ears reaching to touch the soft and gentle thoughts of our mind.

A reflection of a point in time, a smile or a cry that allows us to captures a glimpse of understanding. The understanding of why and who, to form a impression that becomes a deeply imprinted part of our past.

It is not until we reflect on those imprints of our soul that the reflection becomes a part of us, allowing us to remember, re-live, and to give meaning to the imprint. It is our ability to change the bad to good that gives the imprint its place in our spirit. For when we reflect back in time the bad seems to be less bad, and the good seems to be better.

**Thoughts on why
(Written for Karen)**

As the bright golden dawn of the day touches me with it's warm fingers, I think about what it is that has brought me here. Here to this day, this time, and this life. I reflect back on what it is that I have done and why. For I know what I have done but the why just seems to elude me. As I wonder why, why are things the way they are, and why am I the way I am, I must remember that it's not the why of me that I seek, but the why of time. Why is it that time tends to slip past us like a speck of dust that is briskly swept away from it's place of rest, just to rest again and again. It's roots which seem so deeply buried are not as deep as they seem. So it is the why of my life that I am seeking in the ray of the sun. It is the why I have touched and been touched that I must remember. For the why in me, is the why I have touched those around me, and why they have touched me.

So as the ray's of the sun warm my cheeks, I will always remember that I am because of why I am. The why I am is that I am who I am, and that's me.

Just remember it is a gift to touch and to be touched. You have touched many and that is why you are who you are. That is also why things are so hard sometimes.

Chapter 8: Remembering Five Years Past

Its hard to believe that Alexa is already five years old and that it's been five years since the stroke. I have learned a lot since that first day. It is incredible to think that as I look back to where I was I find comfort in knowing that I have survived not only through the support of my family and friends but through the competition with myself to gain each day. When I look back I am reminded of a conversation that I had with a newer stroke survivor. We were at a stroke meeting when he reacted to my telling someone that sometimes its ok to be sad about who we lost. I had once told him that he shouldn't judge himself by who he was but by the progress since the first day of his stroke. I had told him this because he was competitive like me and it could work for him. I now realize that each person reacts to the stress of stroke differently. What motivates me may or may not motivate you. We have to look at the individual independently of "norm." It's harder for some people to face themselves in light of the new person they have become. I know it took me years to come to grip with the abilities of the new me versus the old one. I have learned that the process of change takes time but with time the process can change.

I have been very fortunate to have a significant recovery. I still have some reading, writing, vision and memory problems but I do not let them keep me from obtaining my goals. I have seen how people treat each other and how some try to make themselves feel good by putting others down. It's sad to think that as people we find pleasure in others pain. I smile each day because I have this day and we never know what tomorrow may bring.

When the Spirit Found Me

It was a crisp fall day when my spirit was feeling low that someone inside of me told me where to go. I have no idea why or how he found me but it just happened one day. I have always believed in God but I had never fully understood why. We go through our lives trying to make sense of all of the ciaos when the picture is very clear. I don't remember how the conversation started or why but I do know when it started. It stared the day that Sister Mary had come to the Stroke Group meeting. My church has donated some funds to the group so that we could help others like me. It was then that I decided that it was time to convert from being a Lutheran to Catholic. This may not seem to be such a big deal to some people but to me it was recognition that I truly believed.

My husband is catholic and I made a promise to him that we would raise our children catholic. It was my own conversion that I had not yet recognized. When Sister Mary came to the group and my church so generously donated to help up I realized that it was time. It was time to recognize who I am in a spiritual sense. I have changed so dramatically since the stroke in terms of my knowledge and abilities but I was now beginning to realized that I had also changed spiritually. For quite some time I was angry with God for having put me through all of this. I hated him for it. What I didn't understand was that to heal the spirit had feel and recognize the abandonment it felt. I truly believe that the God in our hearts is good and that he always rests there. When we get lost we push him deeper so that we can't possibly find him. What I know now is that he will creep back into our soul when we let our guard down.

As I gave Sister Mary a hug that day I felt a twinge of hope. It was a feeling I had not had in years. Its like walking though a tunnel to have it open to the warmth of the bright sunshine and the smell of spring. Once she touched my heart it exploded. I craved more of that feeling of satisfaction and contentment. When I walked into church I could feel the change in me.

I talked with my husband about it and he made the call. He told Sister Mary that I wanted to take the necessary steps to convert to Catholicism. He explained my fear of people knowing I couldn't read anymore and my fear of crowds. She assured him that I would be given a sponsor that would be kind and patient with me.

Today was the first day of the rest of my life. I was nervous yet excited about what I would find. I walked into the room with about 15 other people who were there for the same reason. I was introduced to Linda my sponsor and from that day forward I would build a lasting spiritual relationship not only with God but with the Church and her. She was so nice and caring. I was amazed at how comfortable she made me feel. She didn't push me she just talked with me. When I told her my story it touched her. From that point on I found that the burden of stroke seemed a little lighter. I still had bad days but I now have more to look forward too. I looked forward to listing to the stories of the bible and relating them to where I was at that point in time in my life. I search for answers each time I felt his presence. I don't know if others could feel it too but I felt that for the first time in my life I was one of his angels sent to give a message. I was to tell all that we can and do survive and we are as a spiritual people for we have seen what is behind the wall and we have embraced it.

When I walked into the church I could feel his presence touch me. I could see the angels holding me up and lifting me from the crosses that I thought I had to bear. I found sight not with my eyes but with my heart. I felt the passion of people. I felt their sadness. Some would call my sadness liability from stroke I call it insight into who we are to be and how we are to survive. My psychologist gave me the ability to fight for my life and hold on to it but it was the presence of God that helped me fully understand why what had happened to me was not so bad but good. I would have never reached this point in my spirituality at this age had I not had to live through the devastation of stroke. I am not saying that all survivors will find their peace in God because some never will all I am saying is that there is peace after stoke but it is up to you to find it. I found it in the growth of my spiritual self and the new person I am to be and I like that. Some will feel the surge that the church can provide and resist it some will never give it a chance but as long as you know in your heart that you have tried to find peace in your spirit then you have found God. We each must find that place in ourselves that provide us with the our life sight. I have found mine and it rests with God I know that now, I have accepted that, and I truly treasure it.

At the end of the process of conversion we had a party. To celebrate the newness of our spirit I wrote a song. I can't remember the song in its entirety so I have tried to remember as much as I can and add the strength of stoke survival to it. It is not the song itself that matters but the words that it brings. The words I wrote mean a great deal to me I hope that in some way they provide some meaning for you.

Spirit Lost

I was lost in direction
I felt an urgent need.
To feel love and peace and courage.
To feel you presently.

Through you spirit God gave me wisdom.
From those who've seen before.
The strength to say yes lord, I believe in your grace.

I don't see, nor feel you always.
But I'm not like you.

Through you wisdom God gave me meaning.
To help me see the light.
Though my stroke, I found a courage that I had never seen.
So I thank, my lord and family, for strength to be seen.
Please just one gentle moment to hug your neighbor.
For we never know what lays ahead for tomorrow, is never seen.
Be proud of who you are now, not just who you've been.
For we've seen more than most have and we learned to be "me."

Instilling Change

I have instilled in my children that everyone is equal. That no matter how a person looks walks talks and acts that each person deserves to be heard. It's hard to think back and remember that people are cruel and that we often lash out at others because of our own insecurities. I was very insecure when I had my stroke. Learning to like the new me was one of the hardest things I had to do. I look at the stroke as an opportunity to learn. I have learned more than any one person deserves. I have been blessed more than most and realized that if I am to fulfill the promise that I made to my recovery years ago that I had to share my story. Each person has a story. Some stories are good and some stories are bad but one link between all the stories is that they change the heart. The change is proof that our spirits can get us through. I never thought I was a strong person. Now I know that I can survive anything God gives me to bear. I am hoping that I can just foster the hope of one individual to work at recovery the best they can then all of this would be worth it.

I have given of my heart to instill change in people. Taking their burden at times and my own so that they can see what I see. I am but one small person in this life but one thing I do know is that if we each move just one piece of sand with our name on it that we will move mountains as a whole. I am not just one person in this world I am but one of a community of survivors who share a common understanding through stroke that life is not often what it seems but what you make of it.

Change is good. It brings with it new knowledge and understanding. Some changes are harder than others and some we must make whether we want to or not but all change give us the ability to make new decisions and set new direction for that I can see and now understand. So now that I have learned over the past five years I have learned that my story will never be complete because it keeps changing and adding chapters of knowledge and understanding. I don't know what the next five years holds for me but I do know that I look forward to the opportunity to better redefine the new me that would not have been available had I not had a stoke. Like a never ending spiral of hope from all bad can come good and from all good comes knowledge and from all knowledge comes understanding and from understanding come compassion and from compassion comes peace and from peace comes comfort and from comfort comes change.

Chapter 9: Kindness from the heart

After much thought and talking I have decided to end all that I have written here with my thoughts on those people that have cared for me and about me. Out of my heart I asked Christine to read what I have written about, how I felt during the therapy and my recovery from stroke. I do know that what I say and what I do affects others often when I don't realize it. There is a part that I have written and not changed that made her feel as though she was too harsh on me but I know that when I ask I want the truth because I would eventually learn it on my own. I thank her for telling me not what I wanted to hear but needed to understand. She spared me from having to find out on my own through endless failures. The truth gave me the ability to not only understand what had happened to me but to plan for my recovery. I must admit that she was the only person who I would believe when it came to how functional I really was. My family and friends, out of kindness and love, would tell me I was doing well when in fact I wasn't doing as well as I thought I was. Their measurement of my success was not my own. I must comment that my husband, family and friends couldn't have told me how bad I was because I wouldn't have believed them. They have a vested interest in me. It had to come from someone who didn't know me from before. I think I pushed her mentally and spiritually as a therapist and as a human being with a kind heart. As patients we often forget that our teachers are people just like us with feelings. They have chosen a career to help people like us to grow and overcome our stroke deficits. I know that I often did not tell those who helped me the most how much I appreciated what they did for me. I owe my life to my husband, sister, and family, to Christine, Karen and to all those that had a kind word, hugs when I cried, and prayer for my recovery. Without each and every

When I Learn . . .Surviving Stroke with Pride

one I could not have gotten where I am now. I am the only one that can work at recovery but so much of my recovery depended on the people that helped me achieve it.

So what have I learned? I have learned that we often steal the hearts of those that care and never thank them for giving us a part of them to hold on too when we needed it the most. Some days I needed a hug others a kick in the rear without all of these things I would not have learned what I have so graciously learned about life, love and me. Each time I look back I pray that all those that surrounded me with hope know that I too have prayed that they received a part of my heart.

So to all you caregivers, therapists, prayer senders and people with kind heart "thank you" for who you are and for helping me. I may not ever be who I was once before but now I am glad for I am a better person for having lived through stroke. Try not to get lost in the daily routine of the words that we may use for we often forget the impact we can have on you. It is not until we have learned that we fully appreciate what you have given us. "Thank you, from my heart to yours"……Donna

About the Author

Donna L. Brady was born in Las Vegas Nevada in 1963. She is the daughter of Mr. & Mrs. James Jump of Chattanooga TN. Donna's dad served in the USAF for 21 years. Donna has one sister named Karen. Donna traveled extensively a result of her father's USAF career. She played softball for the University of Missouri-Columbia for two years and acted as a Head Counselor during her college summers at Camp Thunderbird for girls located in Northern Minnesota. Donna has a bachelor's degree in Child and Family Development from the University of Missouri-Columbia. Donna was attempting to get her masters degree in Accounting at Walsh College in Troy Michigan when she had her stroke. Donna is happily married to Mr. Mike Brady of Mt. Clemens, MI in August 1987. Mike and Donna have three beautiful daughters who are the focus of their lives. Donna has been working as a contract specialist or procurement analyst for the same employer for the past 16 years.

Donna have survived several traumas in her life, they include:
- Death of a high school classmate from an brain aneurysm,
- An undiagnosed neuralgic event that put her in the hospital for two weeks with full recovery after the birth of her second child.
- Emergency fusion in her cervical spine between C4-5 due to blown disk causing spinal cord compression,
- Stroke six days after the birth of her third daughter, and
- Second cervical fusion about eighteen months after the stroke.

Donna's ability to keep and show a positive attitude has contributed to her recovery. Someone told her, "You are an inspiration to all those that get sick," "your strength to survive and your determination are amazing," and "I look at you and it reminds me of how good life can be." These words inspired Donna to try to write about her stroke and recovery from stroke hoping that she can help others who are trying to survive.

Donna wrote, "That brief conversation from someone I barely know has helped to keep me focused on recovery. If I can just help one person see through the bad to the good, then all this was worth it."

Printed in the United States
60062LVS00001B/142-408